Traumatic Injuries of the Knee

E. Carlos Rodríguez-Merchán
Editor

Traumatic Injuries of the Knee

Springer

Editor
E. Carlos Rodríguez-Merchán
Madrid
Spain

ISBN 978-88-470-5853-8 ISBN 978-88-470-5298-7 (eBook)
DOI 10.1007/978-88-470-5298-7
Springer Milan Heidelberg New York Dordrecht London

Printed on acid-free paper

Springer is part of Springer Science+Business Media (www.springer.com)

Preface

The subject of traumatic injuries of the knee joint represents an important clinical problem. Millions of surgeries are performed every year in attempts to treat traumatic knee injuries. While many treatment options are currently available to orthopaedic surgeons, we need to know which ones are the more adequate to afford the long-term preservation of a fully functional knee.

As such, we have revised the strategies that can restore full knee function both in the short term and in the long run. Therefore, we have assembled a series of chapters that explore and update the diagnosis and treatment of the most important traumatic injuries of the knee joint.

E. Carlos Rodríguez-Merchán

Contents

Distal Femoral Fractures

1

Julián Fernández-González, Santiago J. Ponce, Ruben Fole and Fernando Blanco-Ortiz

1.1 Introduction

According to different opinions, distal femur fractures are located within 7–15 cm from the joint space. It consists of a metaphysis area which is a transition zone between the cylindrical diaphysis and rhomboidal intercondylar area. The two condyles are separated by a depressed longitudinal articular surface, which is the femoral trochlea that articulates with the two facets of the patella. In the posterior aspect, condyles are separated by the intercondylar notch.

The diaphyseal axis has an angle of 6–9° of valgus with respect to the joint line. In the lateral plane the femoral diaphysis continues with the anterior part of the femoral condyles, the ones that extend posteriorly. The condyles in cross-section have a trapezoidal shape which decreases its width from posterior to anterior.

The powerful muscles of the knee are formed by the quadriceps, hamstring, and gastrocnemius muscles. In supracondylar fractures these muscles explain the tendency of the fragments to displace and the action of the gastrocnemius muscles to displace the distal fragment into flexion in the majority of fractures. Overriding of the fragments may be caused by the combined action of the quadriceps and hamstring muscles. Besides recurvatum of the supracondylar fractures, in intercondylar fractures the condyles could be rotated by the heads of the gastrocnemius.

Irrigation of the knee is supplied by the superficial femoral artery which becomes the popliteal artery when passing from the medial to the posterior compartment. The popliteal artery gives the medial and lateral geniculate arteries, whose superior and inferior branches are responsible for the vascularization of both condyles. The lateral femoral condyle is irrigated by superior and inferior lateral arteries, while the medial condyle is irrigated only by the superior medial artery as it passes in front of the medial epicondyle. This is an issue to consider when performing medial knee approaches [1].

1.2 Epidemiology

When proximal femur fractures are excluded, distal fractures represent 30 % of the femoral fractures. They can be caused by high-energy or low-energy trauma [2].

High-energy fractures are generally seen in young patients, these being comminuted, multiplanar, and intraarticular fractures. Among high-energy fractures are the unicondylar (Fig. 1.1) and gunshot fractures (Fig. 1.2). Some of these could be open fractures that increase the severity of the injury.

Low-energy-induced fractures occur on osteoporotic bone, usually in elderly patients, which result in comminuted and multiplanar fractures.

J. Fernández-González (✉) · S. J. Ponce · R. Fole · F. Blanco-Ortiz
Department of Orthopaedic Surgery, Hospital Universitario La Princesa, Diego de León 62, 28006, Madrid, Spain
e-mail: julfergon@hotmail.com

E. C. Rodríguez-Merchán (ed.), *Traumatic Injuries of the Knee*,
DOI: 10.1007/978-88-470-5298-7_1, © Springer-Verlag Italia 2013

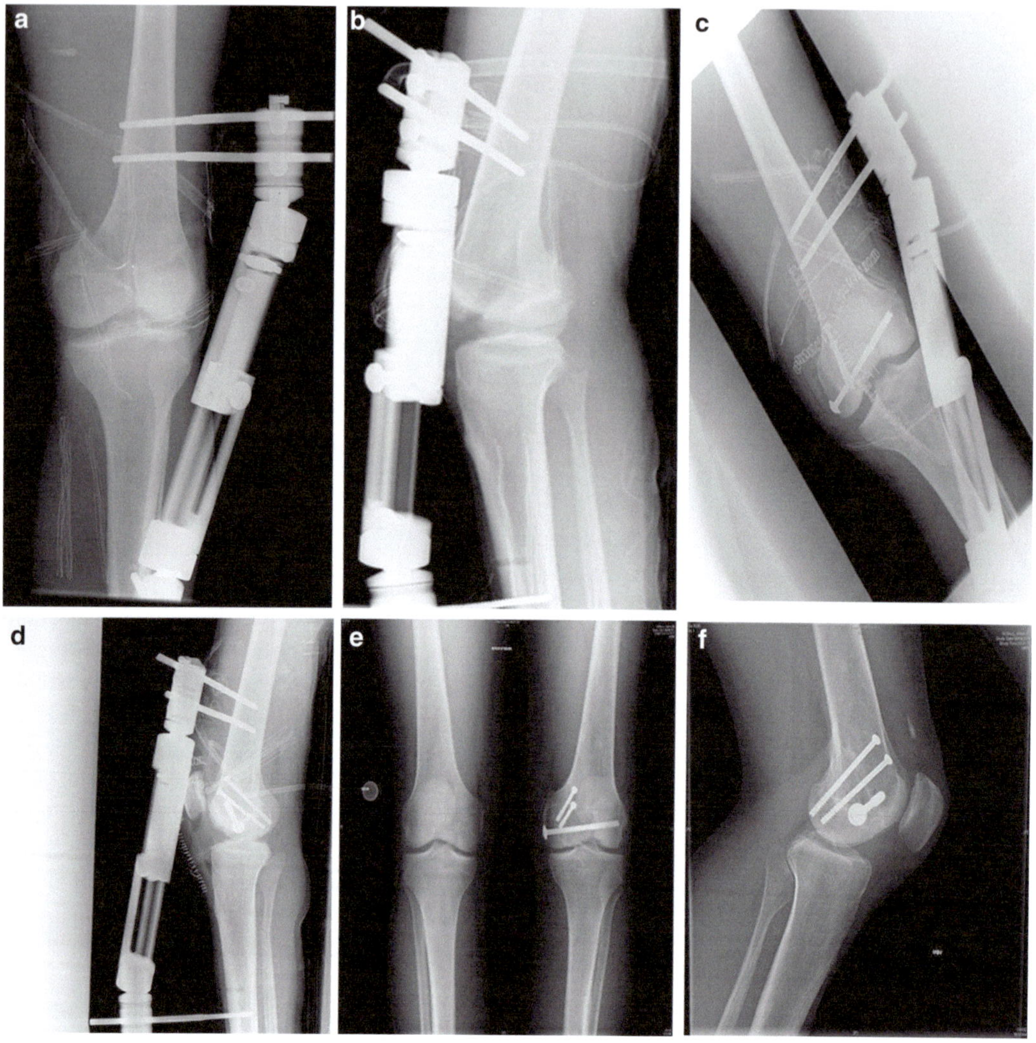

Fig. 1.1 22-year-old patient who suffered a car accident. At the Emergency Unit he was diagnosed of fracture–dislocation of his left knee associated with anterior soft tissue disruption that included a complete ruptured of the quadriceps tendon (**a**, **b**); an early and complete débridement with irrigation fluid, the administration of antibiotics, and a closed reduction of the fracture–dislocation was done and then an external fixator was applied to stabilize the medial unicondylar fracture. One week later, the complex medial unicondylar femoral fracture with two fracture planes was reduced and fixed with three cannulated screws (two for the Hoffa fracture and one for the sagittal fracture) (**c**, **d**). At the same surgery a quadriceps tendon reinsertion was done with transosseous sutures. X–rays done 2 years later showed anatomic restoration of the femoral articular surface, and the patient achieved a good clinical result (complete range of motion), although he needed an open soft tissue release 6 months after open surgery for knee stiffness secondary to quadriceps adherences (**e**, **f**)

Most are produced after falls from a standing position with the knee flexed. However, it is also common to see spiral fractures or fractures with a third butterfly fragment, caused by a torsional mechanism. Often, these patients in addition to osteoporosis carry multiple medical comorbidities and even walking problems.

Medical problems can increase the number of complications, from those related to the fracture as soft-tissue compromise or bone nonunion to general complications which hinder their recovery after a period of inactivity caused by the fracture itself. In these fractures it is important that the patient cooperates in rehabilitation,

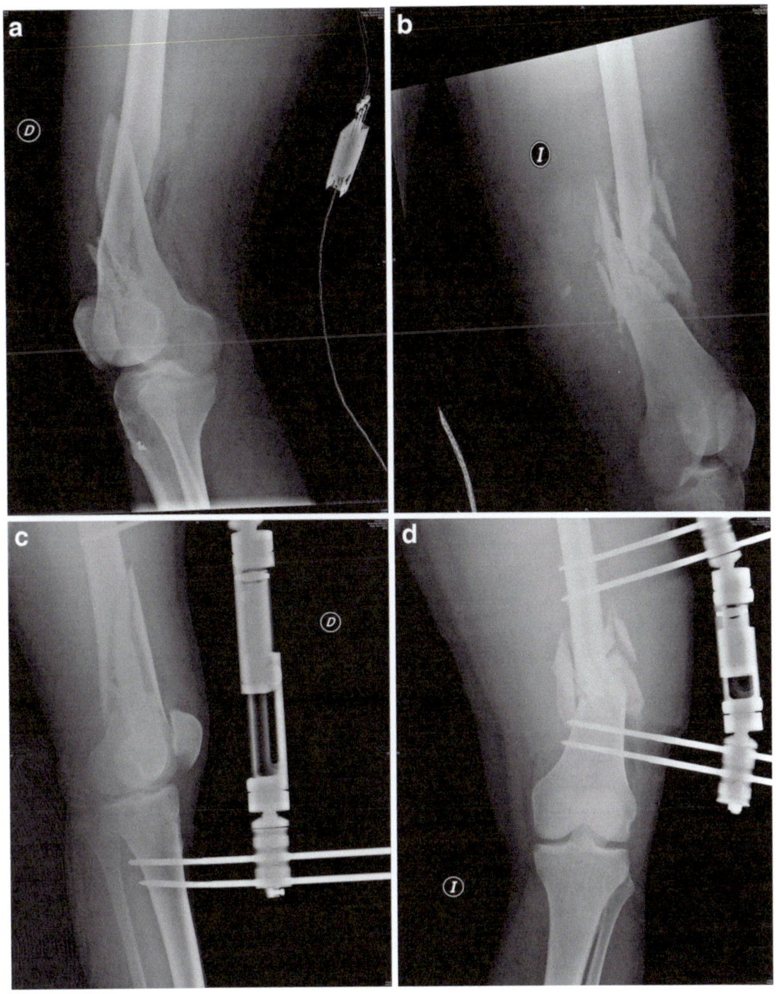

Fig. 1.2 Bilateral distal comminuted supraintercondylar femoral fracture by gunshot (**a**, **b**); external fixation of both fractures was carried out (**c**, **d**); delayed reconstruction was performed once the soft tissues healed

which is greatly affected in patients with cognitive disorders.

An important issue is the fixation of these osteoporotic fractures. Many of these fractures are complicated with early displacement of the fragments which cannot withstand axial and rotational forces.

In young people it is common the association of these fractures with other skeletal injuries, thoracic, abdominal, or head trauma. Always in the emergency area trauma staff should rule out fractures in the same femur at a different level when performing the physical exam and radiological assessment. It is not uncommon the association of ligament injuries in up to 20 % of cases, many of them being diagnosed after the stabilization of the fracture. Vascular injury of the superficial femoral artery or popliteal artery can happen, especially when associated ligament injuries cause posterior dislocation of the fragments. Sometimes, distal femoral fractures can be associated with proximal tibial fractures creating a floating knee, with a high risk of compartment syndrome in that region.

1.3 Classification

There are several classifications for these fractures, but one of the most commonly used is the AO/ASIF classification. Müller et al. in 1991 updated the classification of these fractures and divided them into three groups [3] (Fig. 1.3):

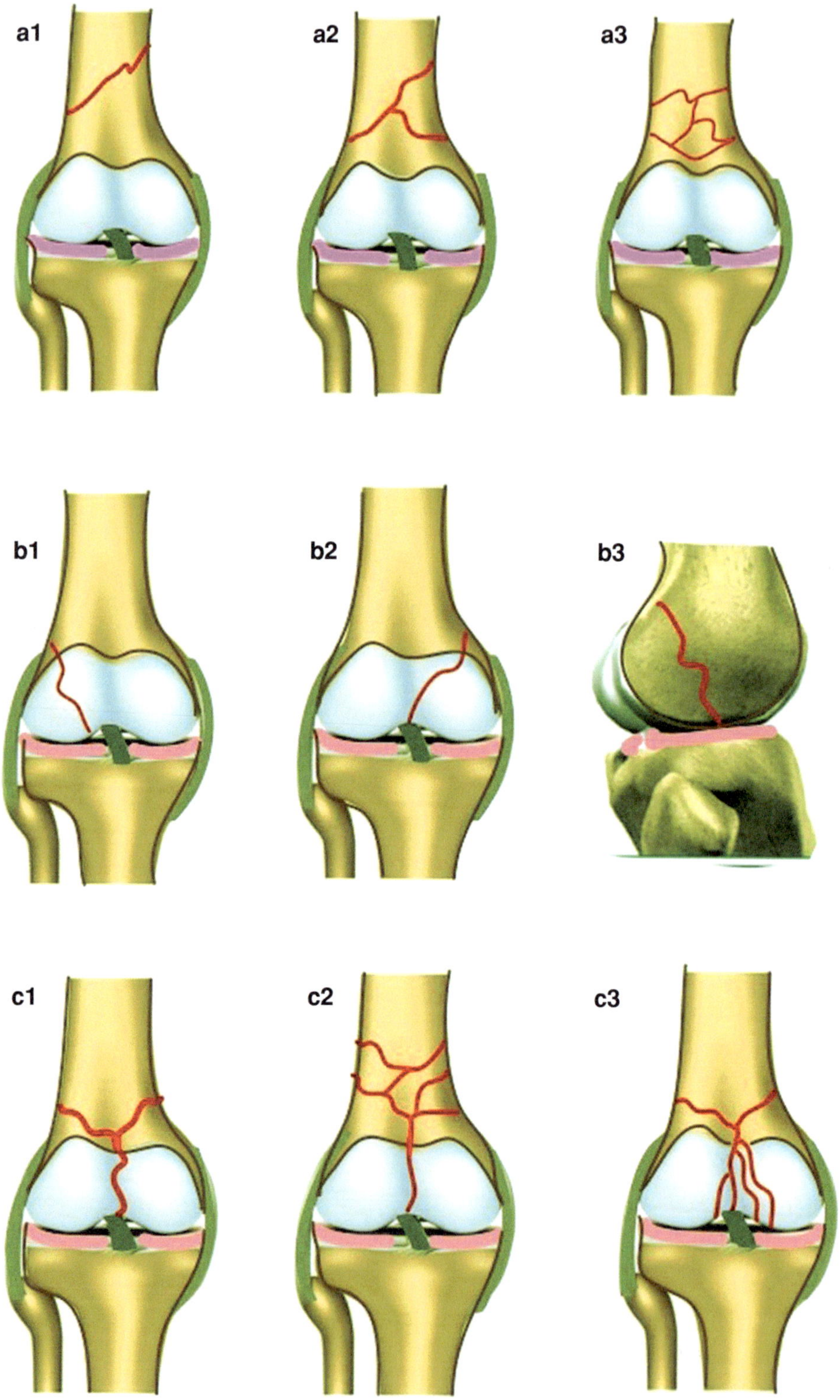

Fig. 1.3 Müller et al. classification of distal femoral fractures [3]

A: Extra-articular fractures
B: Unicondylar fractures
C: Bicondylar fractures.

In turn, these were divided into: A: A1, A2, and A3

- A1: Simple Fracture
- A2: Supracondylar fracture into two parts
- A3: Comminuted supracondylar fracture.

B: B1, B2, and B3

- B1: Fracture of the lateral condyle in the sagittal plane
- B2: Fracture of the medial condyle in the sagittal plane
- B3: Fracture of the lateral or medial condyle in the coronal plane.

C: C1, C2, and C3

- C1: Not comminuted supracondylar fracture with intercondylar extension ("T" or "Y")
- C2: Comminuted supracondylar fracture with intercondylar extension ("T" or "Y")
- C3: Comminuted supracondylar fractures with comminution into the intercondylar fracture.

This classification tells the severity of the fracture and the energy which caused it, both factors increase from types A to C. The severity also worsens from 1 to 3 adding prognostic information.

1.4 Clinical Findings

Patients arrive at the emergency department on stretchers with inability to walk, significant pain, swelling, and deformity clearly apparent in the region of the knee. Patients with low-energy trauma refer to the inability to stand up after suffering the trauma. High-energy injuries are commonly associated with low consciousness level, abdominal or head trauma.

In both cases, a thorough physical examination should be done. In some cases vascular examination is difficult, needing the assistance of a vascular surgeon who sometimes requires additional studies (Doppler studies). If the patient is conscious, the neurologic examination is easily done. It is important to assess soft tissue injuries, to not miss an open fracture with the consequent impact on the treatment and prognosis.

As in all lower limb fractures, one should be alert in the early hours for the possibility of occurrence of compartment syndrome. Ligament examination is preferably done in the operating room.

1.5 Imaging

Clinical suspicion is confirmed by performing a simple X-ray, including at least AP and lateral view of the whole femur, to rule out proximal fractures. This is useful to assess the existence of previous fractures that affect normal anatomic alignment and configuration, or previous fixation or arthroplasty on that femur. In addition, if there is any suspicion that the fracture has entered the joint, a CT scan with sagittal and coronal reconstructions should be done. Appropriate imaging studies are necessary when planning the surgical treatment.

1.6 Treatment

In most cases surgical treatment is recommended. Conservative treatment is currently done only in nondisplaced or incomplete fractures, especially in cases where the patient's poor medical condition or ambulation situation contraindicate surgery.

Currently there are two types of fixation: intramedullary nailing and locked supracondylar plates, with the possibility of percutaneous fixation. Dynamic compression plates (DCP) and dynamic condylar screws (DCS) are used less frequently when compared with nails and locked supracondylar plates, because the latter offer more advantages for fracture fixation. These implants have made almost DCP and DCS obsolete for the treatment of more complex distal femoral fractures.

As mentioned previously, the situation is different if the fracture occurs in a young patient with good bone quality, than if it occurs in an osteoporotic bone of the elderly.

In osteoporotic bone, the implants to be used are the same as in good quality bone, but we recommend the use of longer implants, intra or extramedullary, to avoid the creation of stress risers in the midpart of the diaphysis, which can cause new fractures in osteoporotic bones. Long implants improve the biomechanical strength of fracture fixation constructs and also protect the entire length of the femur [4, 5].

1.6.1 Patient Positioning and Approach

In all cases a supine position is advisable, with the placement of a supporting pad or a small round bump under the distal thigh, which helps to reduce the fracture, especially the flexion–extension deformity. This pad must be placed in a proximal correct position, because a distal placement will result in an extension deformity [4]. Gentle traction applied to the leg may be necessary to correct valgus–varus alignment.

The surgical approach will depend on the type of fracture and the method of fixation. The implant to choose will depend on the type of fracture and the surgeon's preference.

The use of locked supracondylar plates requires a lateral approach with arthrotomy to assess the existence or not of articular fracture lines. Regarding the type of implant and fracture type, incision is extended proximally or not, depending on whether the plate is placed percutaneously or not. Intramedullary nails will require an anterior approach medial to the patellar tendon or through it.

Distal femoral fractures can be divided in extra-articular and intra-articular fractures regarding treatment:

1.6.2 Extra-Articular Distal Femoral Fractures

When we decide on what implant to use, as mentioned previously, now there are two prevalent possibilities: retrograde intramedullary nail and locking compression plates. Each system has advantages and disadvantages.

Retrograde Intramedullary Nail

Conducting intramedullary nailing has the advantage of an indirect approach to the fracture site, respecting soft tissue and hematoma, which will facilitate the fracture consolidation. As mentioned previously, a small approach is necessary.

A complication associated with nailing is malalignment of the fragments. This can be promoted either by an incorrect entry point, or by difficulty to handle the distal fragment during the reaming or nail insertion, which produces extension–flexion deformity of the fracture. To place the nail it is necessary to flex the knee, and with this maneuver the distal fragment generally flexes. It is tempting to make the entry point more posteriorly to avoid that deformity, but it produces anterior translation. The placement of a supporting pad under the distal thigh helps to avoid this complication [4].

The recommended entry point must be 6–8 mm anterior to the posterior cruciate ligament and slightly medial to the center of the intercondylar groove [6]. An incorrect entry point (anterior or posterior) leads to malalignment in the sagittal plane while too medial or lateral, malalignment in varus or valgus [4].

The entry point is undoubtedly the most crucial step. In many cases the use of a C-arm helps in choosing the entry point, despite the intraarticular direct vision with the approach.

Locking Plates

They have a better biomechanical behavior regarding the fixation of the distal fragment, and hence on the stability. In patients with osteoporosis it is advisable to place a longer plate, without placing all the screws on the diaphyseal area [7]. This improves fixation of the bone and bypassing the mid-diaphyseal area reduces the likelihood of fractures in this area by a stress-riser effect, recalling the normal anterior curvature of the femur (Figs. 1.4 and 1.5). Plates are designed to be placed percutaneously and achieve a sufficient length to avoid this potential danger.

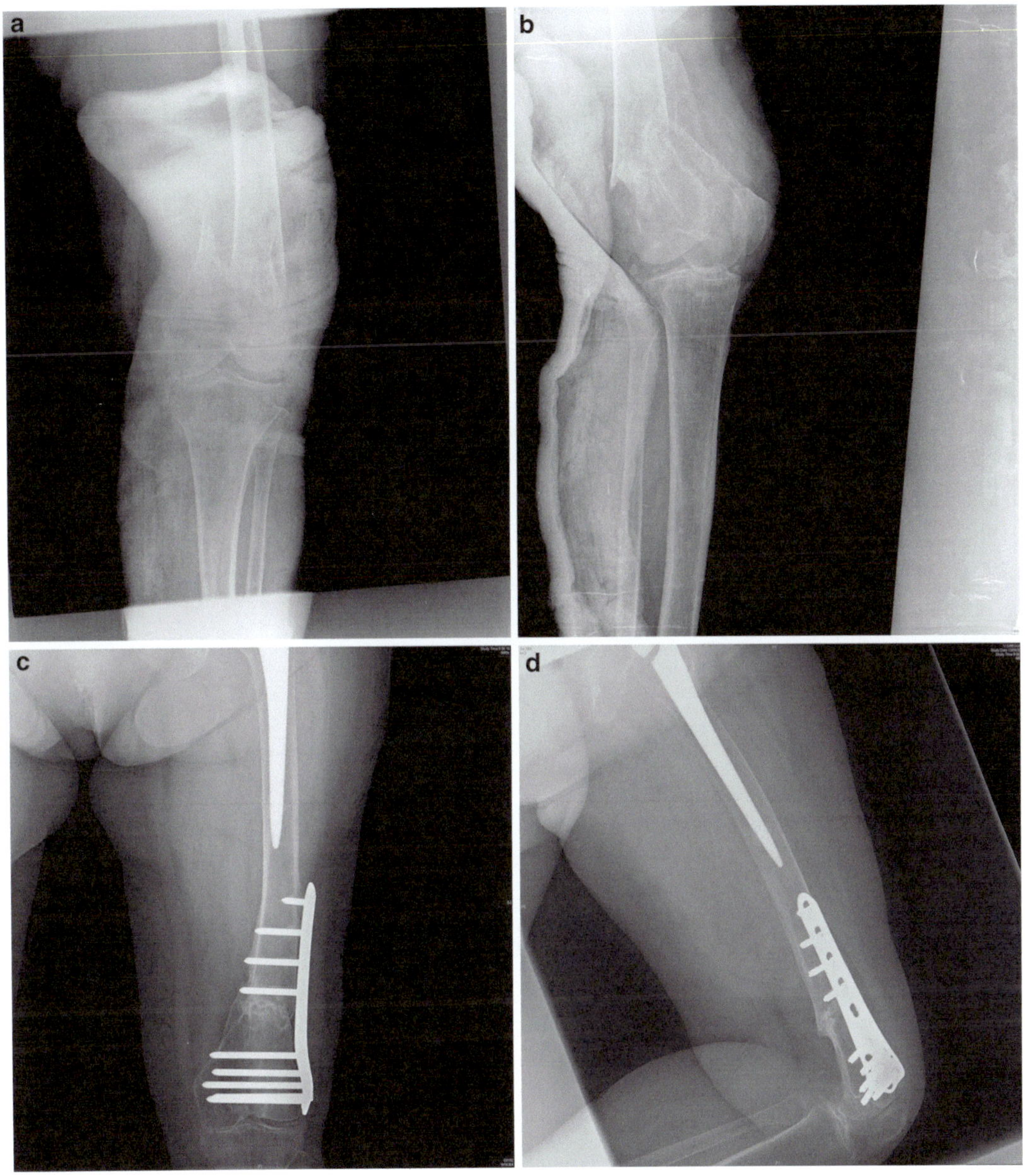

Fig. 1.4 Patient who suffered a supra-intercondylar femoral fracture after a fall. It is interesting to note the existence of a bipolar prosthesis performed several years ago after a displaced ipsilateral intracapsular proximal femur. Posteroanterior and lateral views of the distal femoral fracture (**a**, **b**). X–rays show bone consolidation of the femoral fracture and good alignment in all planes, but probably, the LISS plate should be reached the level of the arthroplasty to avoid stress-riser areas (**c**, **d**)

However, these percutaneous plates have their complications as loss of reduction and failure of the hardware [8]. Although they have shown a biomechanically better performance than traditional methods of fixation (DCP and DCS plates) their placement is not always easy. Prior reduction of the fracture is mandatory before its placement, which is not always easy to achieve. Some authors believe that this technique requires an important learning curve to get good results [9].

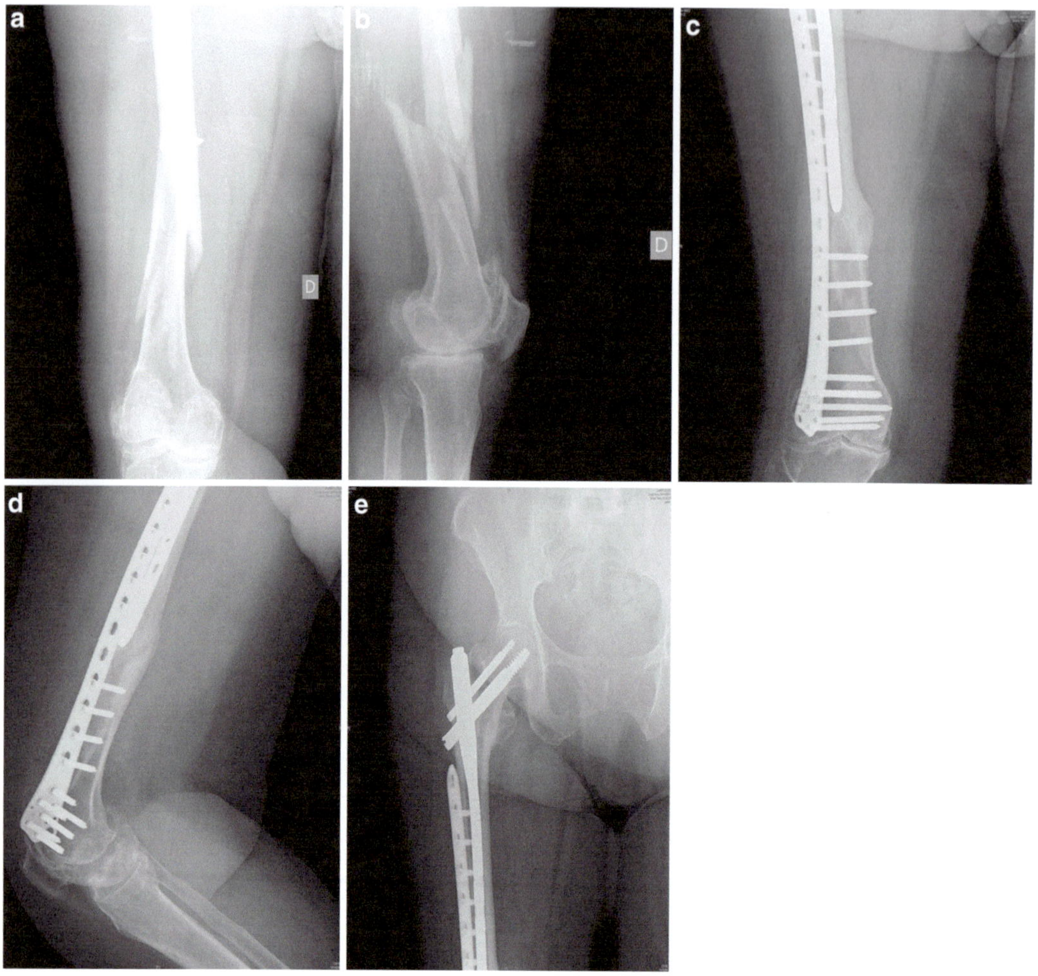

Fig. 1.5 This patient had an extracapsular proximal femoral fracture treated with an intramedullary nail (**a**, **b**). One year later, a supracondylar femoral fracture with proximal extension to the tip of the nail occurred after a casual fall. One year following distal femoral fracture fixation with a locked plate (LISS plate, Synthes^{R}) (**c**–**e**), X–rays showed bone consolidation of the fracture, and good alignment. In this case the locked plate reached the level of the intramedullary device to avoid stress-riser areas

There are reports of screws loosening; to avoid this, the authors of these studies have recommend to avoid early weight-bearing until the fracture is united and to use bicortical screws in most cases of osteoporosis or when there is a reasonable doubt of the risk of nonunion [8, 10]. Also, there have been reports of broken plates, therefore, it is recommended to delay weight-bearing until fracture healing takes place [2, 8–10].

There are facts in favor of plating where infection cases were lower than expected. Probably, extraperiosteal percutaneous placement of the plate entails less soft tissue dissection and periosteal removal of bone fragments on the fracture, which produces less blood loss [11].

As with intramedullary nailing, the placement of plates demands the correct reduction of the fracture avoiding varus–valgus and flexion–extension malalignment.

In cases of severe comminution on the medial side, especially in osteoporotic bone, it is preferable to accept a small shortening of the limb, to achieve the greatest contact of the ends of the fracture and not leave a medial gap. Conversely, in young people with bone discontinuity on the medial side, the application of bone graft or placing another plate on the medial side is recommended, to avoid the risk of varus which frequent occurred in conventional non-locking plates. There are concerns whether locking plates require grafting or an additional plate on the medial side [4].

1.6.3 Intraarticular Distal Femoral Fractures

These fractures are challenging both in osteoporotic bone and normal bone. These fractures have common goals: first, reduction of the intraarticular fracture, second, proper alignment with the proximal fragment, and third, achieve enough stability to allow early motion.

A special situation is unicondylar fractures, which are rare, usually due to high energy. Sometimes, they can be fixed percutaneously, however, to achieve anatomic reduction, open reduction is preferable to restore joint integrity. Usually the fracture fixation with large fragment cancellous screws is enough. Biomechanical studies have shown that placing two large fragment screws is recommended [12]. Sometimes it is necessary to place a plate or more screws when there are more fragments within the fracture.

In supra-intercondylar fractures, after reducing the fragments that form the articular surface, restoring the alignment of the distal femur in all planes is necessary.

In osteoporotic bones, it is possible that there is impaction of the joint surface, which is difficult to reduce, and 1–2 mm of articular surface impaction is acceptable. Disimpaction, in order to recover and maintain the curved form of the articular surface is difficult. The decision will depend on each patient to be treated. In these cases, it is recommended a long locking plate rather than an intramedullary nail [4].

The major problem of osteoporotic fractures is loss of reduction of the distal fragment, even though there is screw placement out of the plate in some cases. Therefore, in cases where fracture stability does not allow early mobilization, consider a knee brace. If the brace or a cast is insufficient, a bridging external fixation may be used. The fixator must be placed in neutral position to protect the locked plate construct. The fixator is removed after 6–7 weeks [4].

1.7 Periprosthetic Fractures of the Distal Femur After Total Knee Arthroplasty

This is an increasingly clinical situation because of the large amount of knee replacements that are done and this is expected to increase in the near future. The ones occurring on the femur are more frequent than those at the tibia. Periprosthetic fractures of the femur are the third most common reason for revision surgery after total knee arthroplasty (TKA), following instability and aseptic loosening.

Risk factors involved in periprosthetic fractures are derived either from the patient itself: advanced osteoporosis, debilitating diseases, inflammatory arthritis, coordination problems; or those derived from the implant: the penetration of the implant in the anterior femoral cortex and excessive osteolysis around the implant. Most periprosthetic fractures are associated with low-energy trauma [13].

Treatment has evolved, so most require surgical treatment, and only those undisplaced or impacted and therefore stable, or those that occur in a patient with significant medical conditions, would require nonsurgical management. In the nonsurgical group is important to assess the risk of general (thromboembolic episodes, bedridden derived complications) and local (joint stiffness and impairment in fracture healing) complications.

The most common situation is an elderly patient with a total knee replacement with good function and no radiographic signs of loosening, with a displaced fracture. Less commonly is a fracture with loosening of the femoral component (Rorabeck and Taylor classification) [14] (Table 1.1).

Table 1.1 Rorabeck and Taylor classification of periprosthetic fractures of the distal femur [14]

Type I	Prosthesis stable, fracture nondisplaced
Type II	Prosthesis stable, fracture displaced (most common)
Type III	Prosthesis loose

In a well fixed implant reduction and stabilization of the fracture should be done. The aim will be to achieve fracture union, maintain limb alignment, length, and rotation.

Fracture type and the medical conditions determine whether fixation is done with a plate or a retrograde intramedullary nail. This will depend on the degree of osteoporosis, comminution of the fragments, the existence of areas of osteolysis, the correct position of the implants, and the presence or absence of a central stem. Each fixation system has its own advantages and disadvantages which are explained below.

When there are radiological signs of loosening of the femoral or tibial component, and if the patient's condition allow, a revision surgery in recommended, with or without associated fixation.

1.7.1 Treatment

In type II cases of Rorabeck and Taylor classification (prosthesis stable and fracture displacement) [14].

Retrograde Intramedullary Nailing

Retrograde intramedullary nailing has shown good results in the treatment of comminuted fractures (Fig. 1.6). Its main advantage is avoidance of further injury to the soft tissue, while providing sufficient stability. The approach is conditioned by previous surgery and type of existing implant. A posterior stabilized (PS) implant will prevent access to the medullary canal. It is indicated in fractures with a cruciate-retaining (CR) implants which preserves the PCL. Bone should be good enough to place two screws with sufficient purchasing to the bone. When there is medial bone comminution or gap, nailing is more stable than the plating, whenever there is adequate distal fixation [15].

A femoral implant not properly placed in medial–lateral direction may condition the distal fragment to displace into varus or valgus (Fig. 1.7). If poorly positioned in an anterior–posterior direction the distal fragment could displace into extension–flexion deformity. Therefore, given the suspicion of a malpositioned implant is preferable to review the indication of intramedullary nailing. Another limitation for nailing is bad quality distal bone, which gives poor purchase of the screws. In situations of maximum osteoporosis, to increase the stability of the nail, a poller screw could be used anterior or posterior to the nail to prevent nail movement.

Only in exceptional cases antegrade nailing could be done, but bearing in mind the creation of stress riser areas between the nail tip and the femoral implant.

Locking Plates

As with nails, femoral implant position will determine the placement of the plate. Locking screws provide high stability in the frontal plane. Some of these plates have polyaxial holes for screw placement which help to avoid the central peg of the prosthesis, thus improving the fixation of the distal fragment [13, 16]. The comminuted metaphyseal area should be avoided to prevent periosteal removal to preserve good irrigation [11]. Plates have this advantage, they can be placed percutaneously. However, the risk of plates as mentioned above is the possibility of malalignment, valgus positioning and hyperextension of the distal fragment [17], which can be avoided with the aid of the C-arm in the operating room.

There are several studies that reported good results, one of them observed only 5 % of failures, medical and orthopaedic complications were infrequent and advise to maintain undisturbed the metaphyseal comminution to preserve the vascularity of the fragments [18].

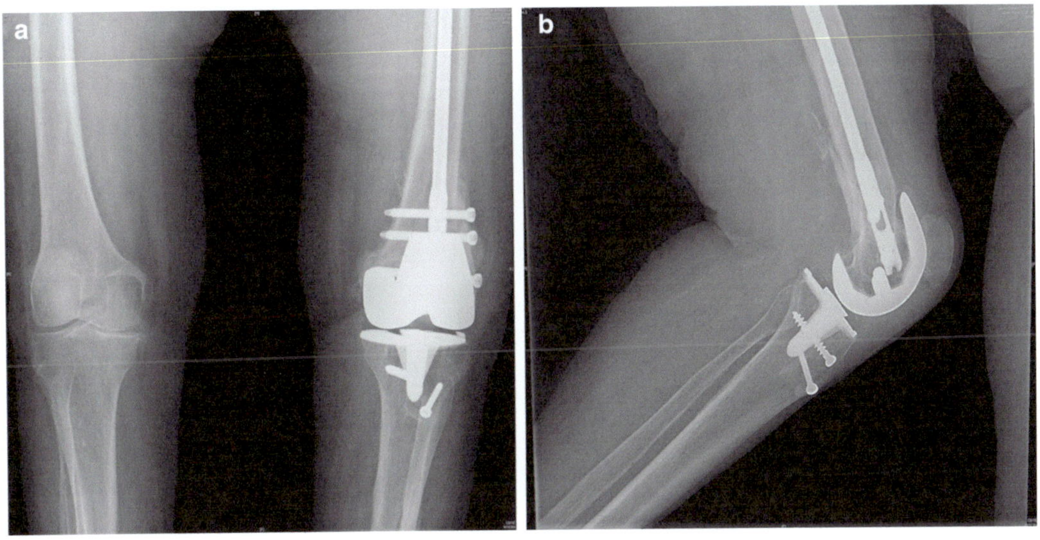

Fig. 1.6 Female patient that underwent a total knee arthroplasty 7 years ago. Two years later, the patient sustained a patellar tendon rupture. An Achilles allograft was used to augment the weak patella tendon suture. Later on, 1 year ago, she fell down and suffered a periprosthetic supracondylar femoral fracture. The periprosthetic fracture was treated with a retrograde intramedullary nail, resulting in bone consolidation with good alignment of the supracondylar fracture (**a**, **b**)

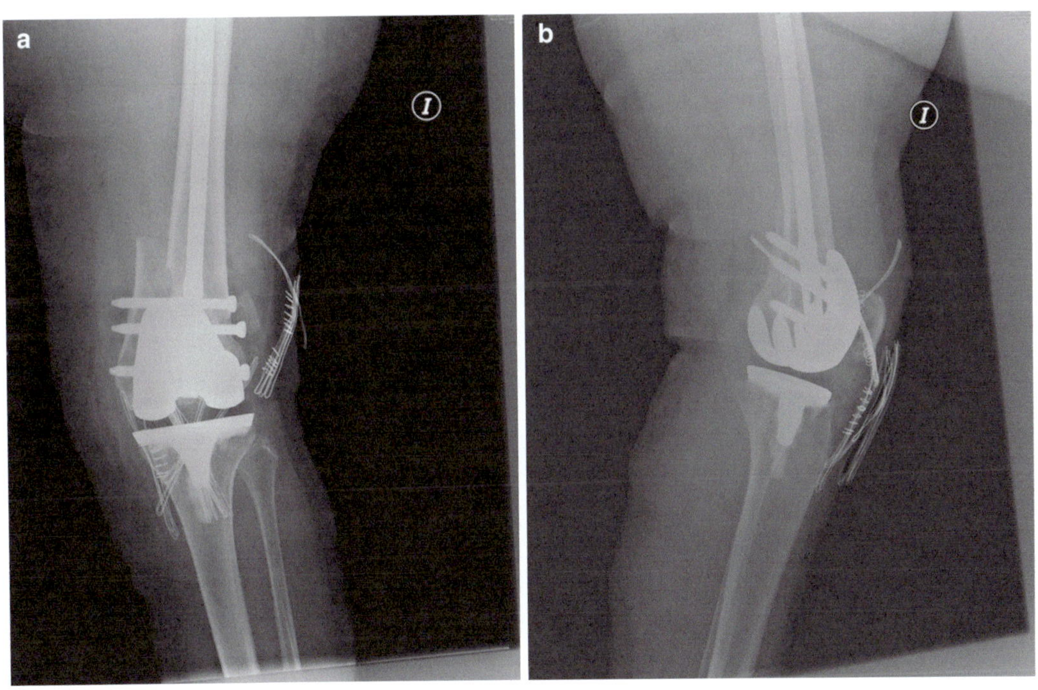

Fig. 1.7 Female patient with many medical comorbidities. She fell down and suffered a supracondylar periprosthetic femoral fracture. She walked with great difficulty and need assistance by her family in the activities of daily life. A retrograde intramedullary nailing was performed. Good alignment was obtained in the sagittal plane but a valgus malalignment was observed in the coronal plane probably due to the position of the femoral component in varus secondary to the difficulty in obtaining a correct closed reduction of these fractures with this technique (**a**, **b**)

1.8 Complications of Distal Femur Fractures

These fractures have a high complication rate. The most common complications are infection, nonunion, malunion, failure of fixation, and stiffness of the knee.

1.8.1 Infection

Infection is one of the most frequent complications. Predisposing factors are high-energy fractures with comminution, open fractures, open surgery with too aggressive periosteal removal, and inadequate fracture stabilization. Thus if there is an articular fracture, reduction should be done and then alignment with the proximal fragment avoiding excessive periosteal stripping. Care should be taken regarding good hemostasis of soft tissue.

Open fractures should be treated properly from the beginning, following an established protocol consisting of extensive irrigation fluid and wound débridement, adequate antibiotic prophylaxis, and followed by temporary or permanent stabilization. Depending on the degree of involvement of the soft tissues, using Tscherne and Öestern classification, a different management will be necessary [19].

If an acute infection develops after fixation of a fracture of the distal femur, the patient should be taken to the operating room and extensive irrigation and débridement of the surgical wound should be done. If the fixation is stable the implant should stay in, whereas when the fixation is inadequate, the material should be removed temporarily and a bridging external fixator should be placed for stabilizing.

In subacute and chronic infections, extensive débridement of the surgical wound should be done, hardware removal and temporary fixation with an external fixator. Upon resolution of the infection, a new fixation should be done if the fracture has not united with the external fixator in place.

1.8.2 Nonunion

It has been seen in operated patients as in patients treated conservatively. Generally, the location of nonunion occurs in the supracondylar area rather than in the intercondylar area.

Factors involved in its development: fractures with bone loss usually many of them are open fractures, fractures poorly stabilized and managed (no grafting in cases of bone deficit), early mobilization, surgical wound infection,and debilitating patient's diseases (diabetes, etc.)

The treatment of nonunion should be addressed to its etiology. In inadequate fixation, proper stabilization and bone grafting should be done. In infected nonunions, irrigation, débridement, and hardware removal must be performed

1.8.3 Malunion

This complication is more common after conservative treatment than after surgery. Malunion could be into varus or valgus in the coronal plane, and shortening or rotational deformity.

After surgery, in supracondylar fractures with comminution on the medial side, a malunion into varus is frequent. To avoid malunion, grafting on the medial side or intramedullary nailing are management options.

It is common malalignment in periprosthetic femoral fractures, in most cases due to an incorrect position of the femoral component.

1.8.4 Fixation Failure

Factors involved are excessive comminution on the fragments in the supracondylar area, a very osteoporotic bone, a very distal fracture that prevents an adequate reduction of the distal fragment and the development of infection.

1.8.5 Knee Stiffness

Knee stiffness is clearly related with a delayed or torpid rehabilitation. Nowadays only a precarious stabilization may contraindicate early active mobilization (within 2–3 weeks). Also an uncooperative patient could be the cause. In these cases the stiffness is due to the development of extraarticular adhesions.

In cases of joint stiffness with an appropriate reduction and stabilization, surgical treatment is more recommended rather than mobilization under anesthesia. It is important and difficult to decide when to mobilize the knee. While the patient keeps improving the range of motion it is advisable to delay surgery. A 6-month period is recommended to wait before surgery, a period where the knee resolves its swelling and an early rehabilitation protocol could be done.

In our experience, surgery should always be open, because if there is not a major articular component in the fracture, adhesions develop in the anterior part of the femur and in major cases of stiffness it develops in the parapatellar recesses that sometimes force the release of ligamentous insertions.

Stiffness may have been caused by an infection and may be responsible for the patient's pain and the difficulty while rehabilitating in the early postoperative period.

1.9 Conclusions

Distal femoral fractures can be caused by high energy or low energy trauma. High-energy fractures are generally seen in young patients, being these comminuted, multiplanar, and intra-articular fractures. The low energy induced fractures occur on osteoporotic bone, usually elderly, which results in comminuted and multiplanar fractures. An important issue is the fixation of these osteoporotic fractures. In most cases surgical treatment is recommended. Currently, there are two types of fixation: intramedullary nailing and locked supracondylar plates, with the possibility of percutaneous fixation. The implant to choose will depend on the type of fracture and the surgeon's preference. Intra-articular distal femoral fractures are challenging both in osteoporotic bone and normal bone. Another issue is periprosthetic fractures of the distal femur after total knee arthroplasty. This is an increasingly clinical situation because of the large amount of knee replacements that are done and this is expected to increase in a near future. Fracture type with a stable prosthesis, the situation most common, and the medical conditions determine whether fixation is done with a plate or a retrograde intramedullary nail. Fractures of distal femur have a high complication rate; that is the reason why we should plan carefully these types of fractures before taking the patient to the operating room.

References

1. Sorkin AT, Helfet DL (2001) Supracondylar and distal femur fractures. In: Insall JN, Scott WN (eds) Surgery of the knee, vol 2. Churchill Livingstone, Philadelphia, pp 1239–1264
2. Schaldenmaier P, Partenhemer A, Koanemann B et al (2001) Distal femoral fractures and LISS stabilization. Injury 32:SC55–SC63
3. Müller ME, Nazarian S, Koch P, Schatzker J (1990) The comprehensive classification of fractures of long bones. Springer, Berlin, pp 116–147
4. Horwitz DS, Kubiak EN (2010) Surgical treatment of osteoporotic fractures about the knee. In: O'Connor MI, Egol KA (eds) Instructional course lectures, vol 59. American Academy of Orthopaedic Surgeons, Rosemont, pp 511–523
5. Zlowodzki M, Williamson S, Cole PA, Zardiackas LD, Kregor PJ (2004) Biomechanical evaluation of the less invasive stabilization system, angled blade plate, and retrograde intramedullary nail for the internal fixation of distal femur fractures. J Orthop Trauma 18:494–502
6. Krupp RJ, Malkani AL, Goodin RA, Voor MJ (2003) Optimal entry point for retrograde femoral nailing. J Orthop Trauma 17:100–105
7. Sanders R, Haidukewych GJ, Milne T, Dennis J, Latta LL (2002) Minimal versus maximal plate fixation techniques of the ulna: the biomechanical effect of number of screws and plate length. J Orthop Trauma 16:166–171
8. Smith TO, Hedges C, MacNair R, Schankat K, Wimhurst JA (2009) The clinical and radiological

outcomes of the LISS plate for distal femoral fractures: a systematic review. Injury 40:1049–1063
9. Schütz M, Müller ME, Krettek C, Hoentzsch D, Regazzoni P, Ganz R, Haas N (2001) Minimally invasive fracture stabilization system of distal femoral fractures with the LISS : a prospective multicenter study. Results of a clinical study with special emphasis on difficult cases. Injury 32:SC48–SC54
10. Button G, Wolinsky P, Hak D (2004) Failure of less invasive stabilization system plates in the distal femur. A report of four cases. J Orthop Trauma 18:565–570
11. Farouk O, Krettek C, Miclau T, Schandelmaier P, Guy P, Tscherne H (1999) Minimally invasive plate osteosynthesis: does percutaneous plating disrupt femoral blood supply less than the traditional technique? J Orthop Trauma 13:401–406
12. Hak DJ, Nguyen J, Curtiss S, Hazelwood S (2005) Coronal fractures of the distal femoral condyle: a biomechanical evaluation of four internal fixation constructs. Injury 36:1103–1106
13. Della Valle CJ, Haidukewych GJ, Callaghan JJ (2010) Periprosthetic fractures of the hip and knee: a problema on the rise but better solutions. In: O'Connor MI, Egol KA (eds) Instructional course lectures, vol 59. American Academy of Orthopaedic Surgeons, Rosemonts, pp 563–575
14. Rorabeck CH, Taylor JW (1999) Periprosthetic fractures of the femur complicating total knee arthroplasty. Ortho Clin North Am 30:265–277
15. Bong MR, Egol KA, Koval KJ, Kummel FJ, Su ET, Iesaka K (2002) Comparison of the LISS and a retrograde-inserted supracondylar intramedullary nail for fixation of a periprosthetic distal femur fracture proximal to a total knee artthroplasty. J Arthroplasty 17:876–881
16. Haydukewych GJ, Sems SA, Huebner D, Horwitz D, Levy B (2008) Results of polyaxial locked-plate fixation or periarticular fractures of the knee: surgical technique. J Bone SJoint Surg Am 90(suppl 2 pt1):117–134
17. Haidukewych GJ (2004) Innovations in locking plate technology. J Am Acad Orthop Surg 12:205–212
18. Kregor PJ, Hughes JL, Cole PA (2001) Fixation of distal femoral fractures above total knee arthroplasty utilizing the less invasive stabilization system (L.I.S.S.). Injury 32:SC64–SC75
19. Öestern HJ, Tscherne H (1984) Pathophysiology and classification of soft tissues associated with fractures. In: Tscherne H, Gotzen L (eds) Fractures with soft tissue injuries. Springer, Berlin, pp 1–9

2 Tibial Plateau Fractures

Juan Carlos Rubio-Suárez

2.1 Introduction

Fractures of the tibial plateau affect a large weight-bearing joint. Hence they are severe and can provide serious functional abnormalities. The main goals of the treatment are to recover the joint congruency and the normal mechanical axis, ensure the stability, and obtain a wide range of motion. To achieve these objectives is very difficult and depends not only on the treatment, but also on the state of the soft tissues, bone quality, and patient age and associated diseases. Tibial plateau fractures are 1 % of all fractures and 8 % in the elderly. The most common are external plateau (55–70 %). Isolated lesions of the medial plateau are between 10 and 23 %; and the fractures affecting both plateaus are 10–30 % [1].

The mechanism of injury can be: (1) A force applied on the lateral side directed medially. The effect is a valgus deformity resulting in a bumper fracture of the lateral plateau; (2) a force applied on the medial side and directed laterally. It produces a varus deformity and a medial plateau fracture; (3) an axial compression force combined or not with a force from the side. In this case, the result is a both plateaus fracture.

However, the fracture pattern also depends on the energy and on the age. In young people, after a high-energy trauma, the plateau is broken into various fragments but the depression of the joint surface is not common. By contrast, the aged low-energy trauma shows the classical bumper fracture. This is a lateral plateau fracture with little or no displacement but with a central depression in the articular surface.

Tibial plateau fractures can be associated with serious soft tissues damage [2] such as tears of the menisci, tears of the collateral, or cruciate ligaments [3]. Moreover, the fractures of the medial plateau are often associated with lesions of the peroneal nerve or the popliteal vessels. High energy fractures are often associated with severe skin damage with edema, bruising, and swelling that affect the time of surgery.

2.2 Diagnosis

It is important to know the characteristics of the injury such as energy, force direction, and deformity produced. It allows us to predict the severity and type of fracture.

2.2.1 Physical Examination

Physical examination provides us information about the state of soft tissues envelope. We must

J. C. Rubio-Suárez (✉)
Department of Orthopaedic Surgery, "La Paz" University Hospital-IdiPaz, Paseo de la Castellana, 261, 28046, Madrid, Spain
e-mail: rubioj57@gmail.com

E. C. Rodríguez-Merchán (ed.), *Traumatic Injuries of the Knee*,
DOI: 10.1007/978-88-470-5298-7_2, © Springer-Verlag Italia 2013

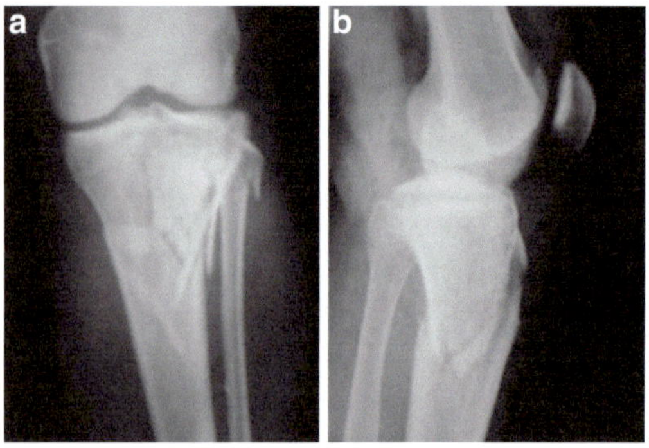

Fig. 2.1 Antero–posterior (**a**) and lateral (**b**) X-ray views of a tibial plateau fracture

not forget to explore the neurologic and vascular status of the limb. Finally, we should evaluate the existence of a compartment syndrome.

2.2.2 Imaging

Standard X-Ray Views

AP and L views must be taken, but are insufficient so we should take oblique projections. These give us excellent information about the plateau state (Fig. 2.1).

CT Scan

Computed tomography (CT) is an excellent diagnostic tool. Three-dimensional reconstruction allows us to know the fracture and to plan the surgery and the surgical approaches accurately [4]. Moreover, if vascular lesion or compartment syndrome is suspected, to perform a CT angiography is mandatory (Fig. 2.2).

Magnetic Resonance Image

Tibial plateau fractures are often accompanied by meniscus and ligament tears. The diagnosis of these lesions must be made on admission. The magnetic resonance image (MRI) study is very useful for that. However, it does not preclude the realization of a CT scan [5].

2.3 Classification

There are many classifications of tibial plateau fractures. However, two of them are the most used nowadays because they are simple, understandable, and useful to establish treatment and prognosis.

2.3.1 AO classification

Tibial plateau fractures belong to the segment number 41. Type A are extra-articular fractures [1] :

- A-1: avulsion of the tibial spines
- A-2: metaphyseal simple fracture
- A-3: metaphyseal complex fracture

Type B fractures affect the joint surface but only one of the two plateaus:

- B-1: simple condylar split
- B-2: impactions with more or less articular surface subsidence
- B-3: combination of split and depression

We add 0.1 when the fracture affects the lateral condyle and 0.2–0.3 if the fracture affects the medial condyle.

Type C fractures affect both condyles with articular and metaphyseal strokes:

- C-1: simple articular and metaphyseal fracture
- C-2: simple articular and complex metaphyseal
- C-3: complex both articular and metaphyseal

2.3.2 Schatzker Classification

It is perhaps the most used today and divides plateau fractures into two groups with three types in each group [6]. The first group includes the low-energy fractures

- I: Simple split fracture of the lateral condyle.
- II: Split and depression fracture of the external condyle.
- III: Central depression in the lateral condyle.

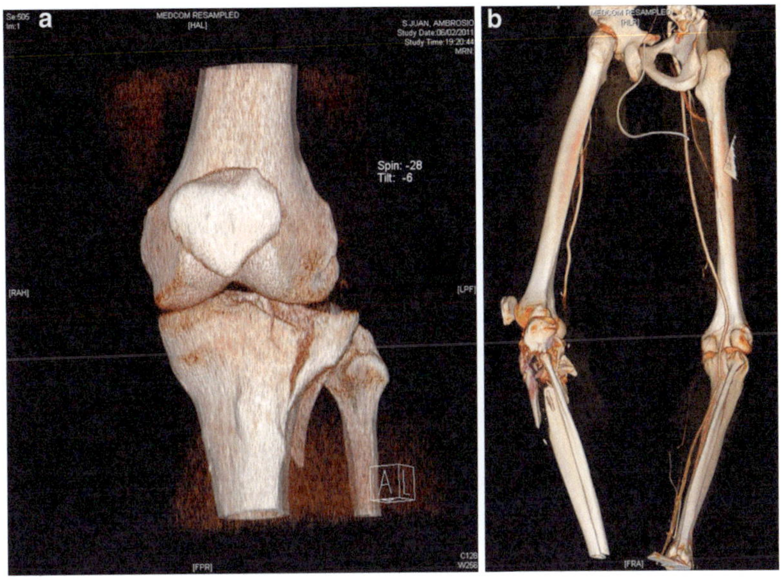

Fig. 2.2 CT scan: (**a**) 3D reconstruction; (**b**) angio CT in complex fracture of proximal tibia with stop in popliteal artery

The second group consists of high energy fractures:

- IV: Fracture of the medial condyle. It is rare but is frequently accompanied by neurovascular injuries (5–50 % peroneal nerve, 13–50 % popliteal artery) and/or compartment syndrome.
- V: Bicondylar fracture without metaphyseal affectation.
- VI: Fracture of both condyles and metaphyseal.

Type V and VI fractures are frequently associated to severe soft tissue injury.

2.4 Treatment

The goal of fracture treatment is to get a stable, congruent, and aligned joint in order to avoid the risk of posttraumatic osteoarthritis and reduce the pain [7]. Factors determining the prognosis are: (1) articular collapse; (2) condylar separation or widening; (3) epiphyseal-metaphyseal dissociation; and (4) soft tissue integrity.

Therefore, a precise anatomical reconstruction of the joint and a stable fixation is required to get an early mobilization and prevent degenerative changes [8]. Mechanical studies have demonstrated that the joint mismatch tolerance is not greater than 1.5 mm [9]. Schatzker, based on those observations, pointed out the following:

1. Articular fracture with instability requires open reduction and internal fixation.
2. The joint congruence can be recovered mean open reduction only.
3. Anatomical reduction and stable fixation is required for cartilage regeneration.
4. If the patient conditions do not allow surgical treatment, the fracture must be treated by skeletal traction and early motion.

2.4.1 Nonsurgical Treatment

The indications of the conservative management are: (1) uncompleted or slightly displaced fractures; (2) stable and slightly displaced fractures of the lateral condyle; (3) severe osteoporotic bone; (4) elderly with little or no functional demand; (5) patients with severe disease and high surgical risk; (6) spinal cord injury patients; and (7) inexperience of the surgeon.

Stable and non-displaced fractures, especially those affecting the lateral condyle, are usually treated by joint aspiration (arthrocentesis) followed by immobilization with cast above the knee for 4–6 weeks. Then we replace the cast by an orthesis for another 4–6 weeks, allowing progressive flexion of the knee until 90° and walking without weight bearing helped by crutches. At 8–12 weeks the progressive weight bearing is allowed to become full.

In unstable, displaced, or comminutes fractures, the management consists of skeletal traction with 4–7 kg mean a pin placed in the supramalleolar region of the tibia, for 4–6 weeks. This will reduce the fracture by ligamentotaxis, but not reduce the sunken fragments, keeping the alignment. During this time flexo-extension movements of the knee are allowed. Between 6 and 12 weeks a hinged brace is placed allowing no weight bearing ambulation. Finally, from week 12 progressive weight bearing ambulation is allowed.

2.4.2 Surgical Management

Surgical management is preferred in most displaced, comminutes, and incongruent fractures. The goal is the anatomical open reduction and internal fixation. A correct and accurate preoperative planning is mandatory. Absolute indications of the surgical treatment are [7]: (1) open fracture; (2) associated acute compartment syndrome; and (3) acute arterial lesion

Relative indications are: (1) fractures of the lateral plateau (types II and III) causing instability; (2) fractures of the medial plateau (type IV) displaced; and (3) bicondylar fractures (types V and VI).

Time of Surgery

Isolated tibial plateau fractures, should be stabilized as soon as possible by means of open reduction and internal fixation. Open fractures, with compartment syndrome or vascular injury must be treated immediately. However, patients with multiple injuries, especially those with head, thoracic, or abdominal injury, must be stabilized provisionally using an external fixator (damage control orthopedics) until the general conditions improve (window of opportunity, 5–10 days after injury). On the other hand, closed fractures with severe damage of soft tissues should not be undergone to open reduction and internal fixation immediately [10]; in such cases we must do a sequential treatment. First, we stabilize the fracture provisionally by means of an external fixator (Fig. 2.3). Once soft tissues are improved, and not before 2 or 3 weeks, we change the external fixator with a final internal fixation.

Definitive Treatment

Preoperative planning

Good preoperative planning helps the surgeon a lot, as it shortens the surgical time, avoids improvisation, and ensures the availability of the necessary resources.

Surgical approaches

Spinal anesthesia is used unless contraindicated. The patient should be on a radiolucent table in supine position. A sterile tourniquet is preferable. Fractures of the lateral tuberosity are approached across anterolateral incision. Medial tuberosity fractures are approached through a posteromedial incision. Both tuberosities fractures could be approached by means of an anterior incision but this approach provides a low vision of the fractures. Therefore, two incisions, anterolateral and posteromedial are recommended, especially in complex fractures [11]. We must take special care to avoid skin necrosis. Straight longitudinal incisions are recommended to avoid damage of the cutaneous vasculature and lift big flaps must be avoided [12] (Fig. 2.4).

The Preferred Treatment for Each Type of Fracture

Type I

The fractures of the lateral condyle without sinking are usually complicated with detachment or tear of the external meniscus [13]. Therefore, it is useful to do an MRI. The preferred treatment is internal fixation (Fig. 2.5). It can be done closed, using percutaneous screws and checking the reduction by means of arthroscopic control. It can also be done by open reduction with direct view of the joint surface and meniscus. Two or

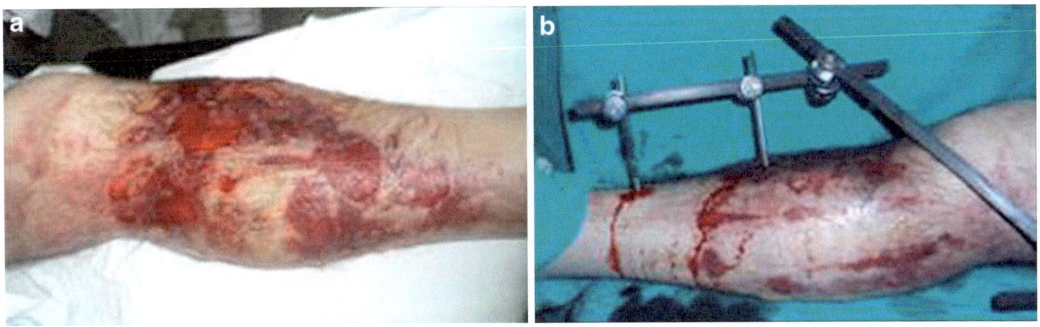

Fig. 2.3 Tibial plateau fracture with severe soft tissue injury (**a**) managed by external fixator (**b**)

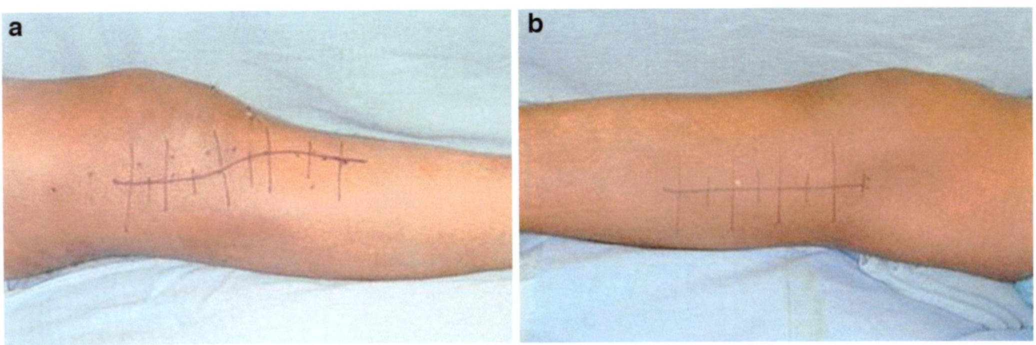

Fig. 2.4 Surgical approaches to proximal tibia. Skin marks: anterolateral (**a**); posteromedial (**b**)

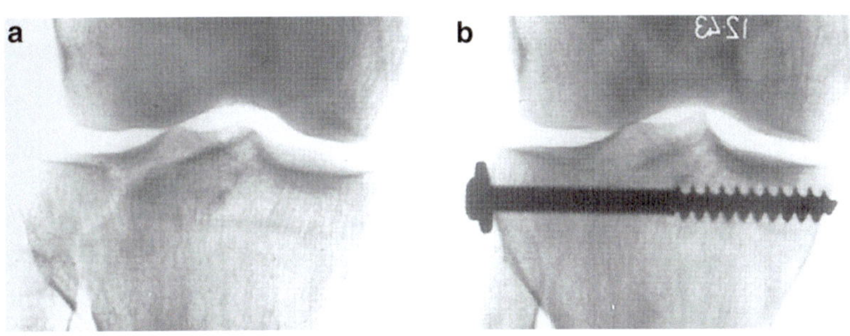

Fig. 2.5 Schatzker I fracture (**a**). Treatment by percutaneous screw (**b**)

three cannulated screws are usually enough to provide stability [14].

Type II
This is a fracture of the lateral condyle accompanied by some degree of collapse of the joint surface. In this case, open reduction under direct vision of the joint is mandatory. The sunken articular fragment must be replaced and fastened with bone graft or bone substitute [15] placed in the vacuum left after replacement. Then, the lateral condyle can be fixed with two or three cannulated screws, though it is better use a buttress plate.

Type III
There is a central sinking in the joint surface but not condylar fracture. It is typical of elderly patients with osteoporotic bone suffering valgus mechanism. We make nonsurgical treatment

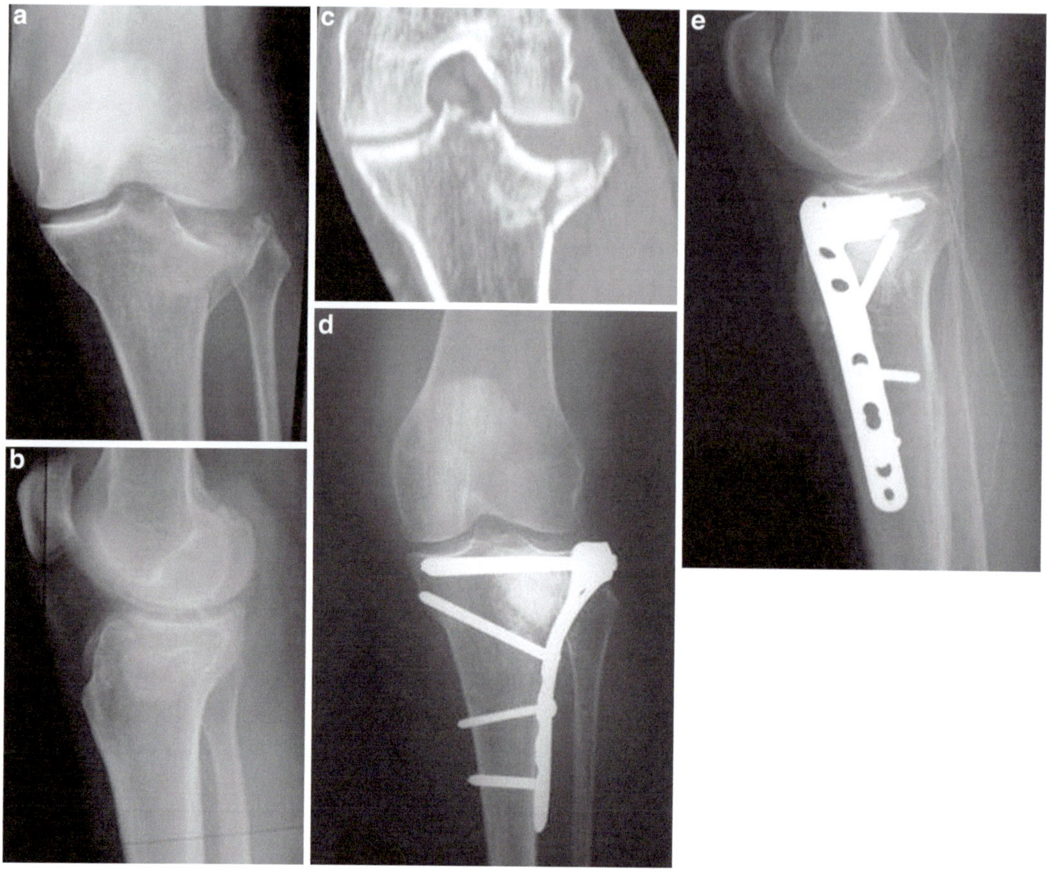

Fig. 2.6 Schatzker II fracture: AP (**a**) and lateral (**b**) X-ray views; (**c**) CT scan image; (**d**) and (**e**) postoperative radiographs. Reduction of the sunk fragment and stabilization of the fracture by means of a lateral plate and hydroxiapatite graft can be seen after surgical treatment

when the collapse is lesser than 2 mm and the joint is stable. Otherwise, we must do surgical management. We should perform a CT or an MRI to determine the amount and location of the sinking. Nowadays surgery can be done by means of minimal invasive techniques (Fig. 2.6). Across a small incision on the skin, a window in the lateral face of the proximal tibia is done to elevate the sunken fragment. The reduction is checked by arthroscopic view [16]. Finally, the vacuum created after the fragment replacement is filled through the bone window with bone graft or bone substitute.

Type IV

This fracture affects the medial condyle (Fig. 2.7) and is often caused by high-energy trauma. There is a high frequency of soft tissues, ligaments, and neuro-vascular injuries associated with these fractures. Surgical treatment is preferred in most cases which is carried out through a medial approach. The medial incision should be as posterior as possible in order to reduce the posterior fragment. A buttress plate is necessary to improve stability after open reduction (Fig. 2.8).

Types V and VI

These fractures affect both lateral and medial tibiae condyles (Fig. 2.9). They are produced by high energy trauma and soft tissue damage is highly frequent [17]. The preferred treatment of these fractures is open reduction and internal fixation through two approaches: anterolateral and posteromedial. Anatomical reduction to restore the joint surface and the limb alignment

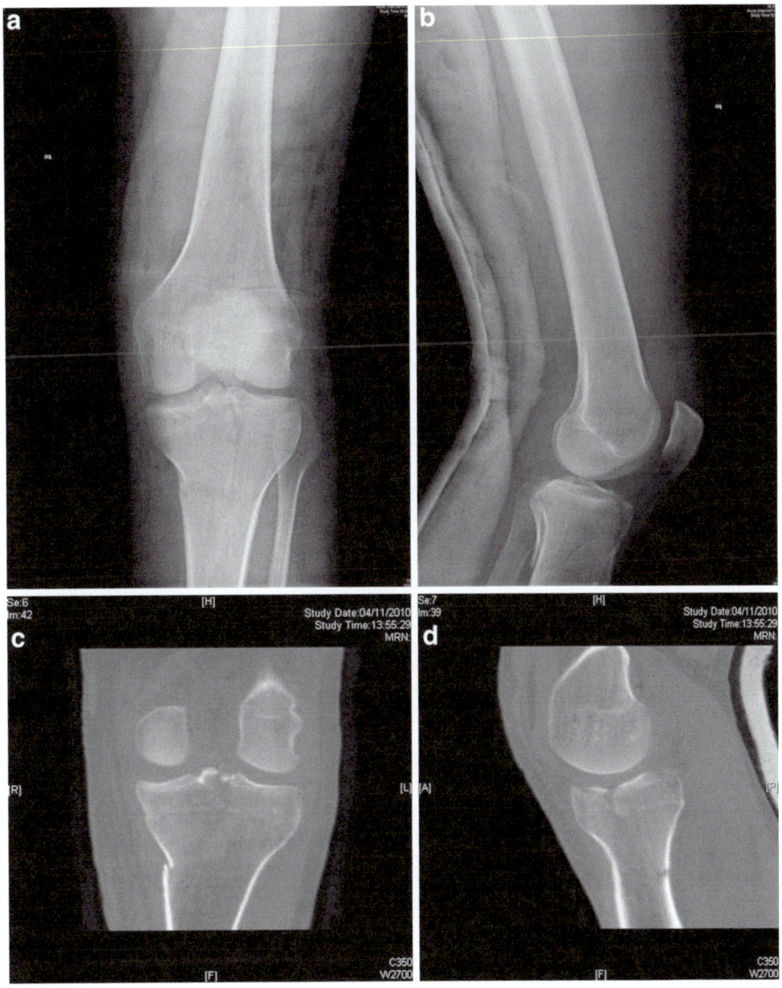

Fig. 2.7 Schatzker IV fracture: (**a**) X-ray views; (**b**) and (**c**) CT-scan images

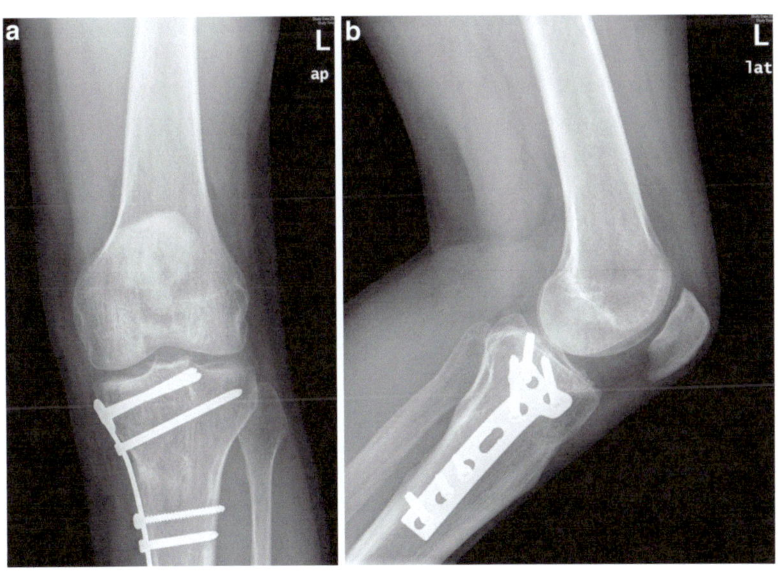

Fig. 2.8 The same fracture as in (Fig. 2.7) with medial osteosynthesis plate: AP view (**a**); lateral view (**b**)

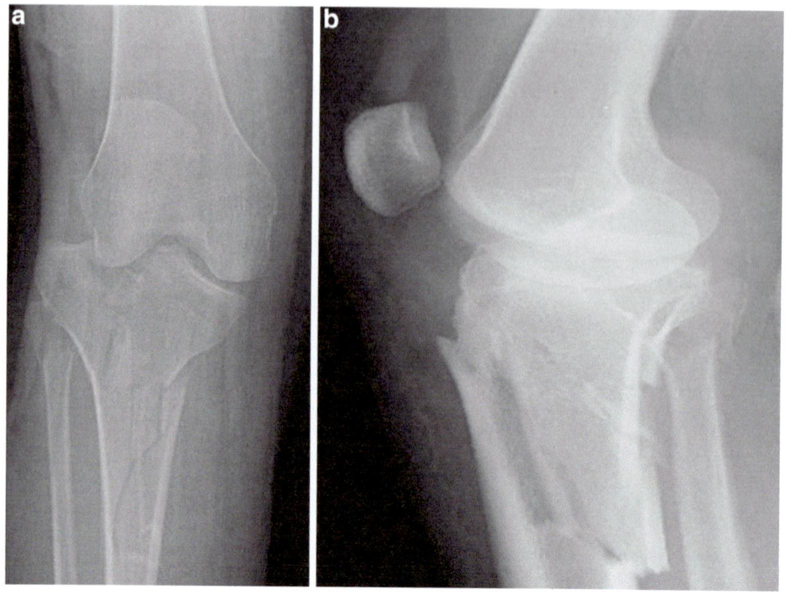

Fig. 2.9 Schatzker VI fracture; AP view (**a**); lateral view (**b**)

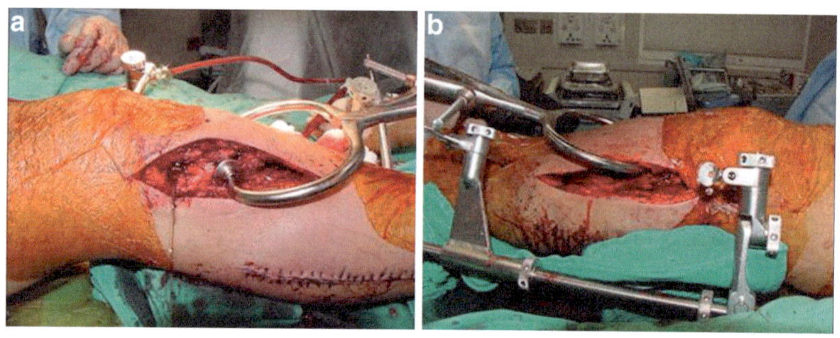

Fig. 2.10 Surgical approaches and instruments for reduction: clamp (**a**) and distractor (**b**)

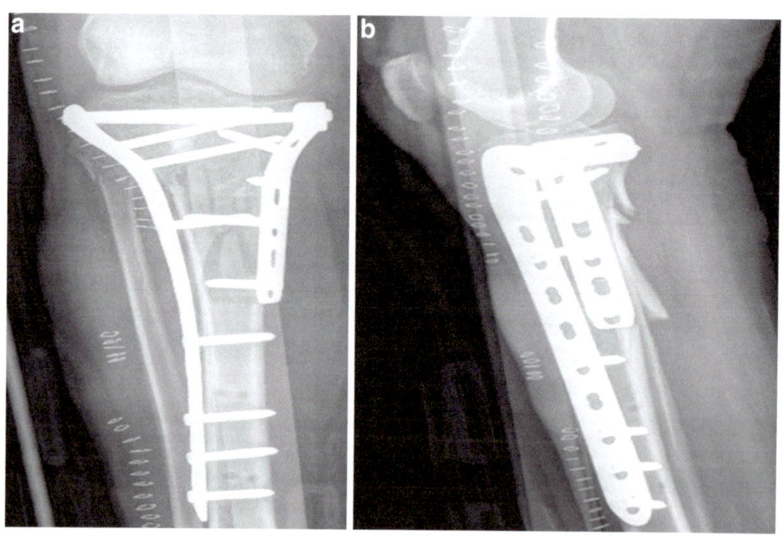

Fig. 2.11 Lateral and medial osteosynthesis plates for Schatzker VI fracture: AP view (**a**); lateral view (**b**)

is mandatory. Many a time it can be helpful to use a distractor (Fig. 2.10); the distraction helps to get the reduction by ligamentotaxis, keeping the fragments in place while the fracture is fixed with plates (Fig. 2.11).

However, the open reduction and internal fixation (ORIF) often complicates by wound dehiscence or infection which may lead to failure of work [5]. To avoid these complications in complex fractures with severe affectation of soft tissues many authors advise the use of hybrid external fixation [18]. The hybrid construction is made with tensile wires and ring in the proximal tibiae and threatened pins in tibial shaft, all of them through percutaneous insertion. The joint surface reduction can be checked by arthroscopic view. The hybrid external fixation can be combined with internal fixation through percutaneous cannulated screws. This minimal invasive method provides good results because it does not add damage to the injured soft tissues [19].

Special Situations

Open fractures

Open fractures of the tibiae plateau are not frequent and are often accompanied by major trauma in multiply injured patient. The management of these fractures requires reflection, experience, and prudence. Washing, wide débridement, and antibiotic coverage are key to the treatment of these fractures. In level 1 trauma centers with skilled surgeons they can be treated with immediate ORIF, whenever early soft tissue coverageis performed. Hence trained plastic surgeons in this kind of injury must be available. Otherwise, a sequential treatment will be more prudent. At first, washing, débridement, and temporary external fixation until the soft tissue has healed are what we must do. The external fixator should bridge the knee placing pins in distal femur and tibial shaft applying the principle of ligamentotaxis. Once the soft tissue is healed (2–3 weeks) external fixator is changed by internal fixation according to the type of fracture.

Vascular injury

Fracture types Schatzker IV, V, and VI are put at risk of injury to the popliteal artery and its three branches. If we suspect arterial injury, arteriography or angio-CT should be done. Arterial injury must be repaired as soon as possible; however, we must first restore both the length and axis of the limb and stabilize the fracture. To do that, we can use an external fixator. The arterial repair is usually done with by-pass using vein graft or Teflon prosthesis. Finally, fasciotomy opening the four compartments of the leg is mandatory.

Ligament injury

Ligament injuries are often associated to tibial plateau fractures. It is estimated that the incidence of these injuries is between 30 and 56 % of all cases [20]. However, many of them go misdiagnosed. Medial ligament was injured in 20 %, lateral ligament in 3 %, and anterior cruciate ligament in 10 % of cases [2]. We should always take study using MRI to diagnose these lesions.

Repair of these lesions should not be done during the initial repair of the fracture. Conservative treatment is recommended at first. When the instability is persistent surgical repair is indicated once the fracture has healed and the hardware has been removed.

2.4.3 Postoperative Treatment

One or two suction drains are left for 2 days and prophylactic antibiotherapy is administered for 24–48 h. When the fixation is stable the main goal is to get a wide mobility of the knee. During the first week the patient can do passive motion till obtaining 90° of arch. Then, he must start with active motion in order to improve the arch of movement and the muscle tone. Weight bearing is not allowed until weeks 6–12, when we check the healing of the fracture [21]. During this time, the patient must walk without weight bearing, helped with crutches.

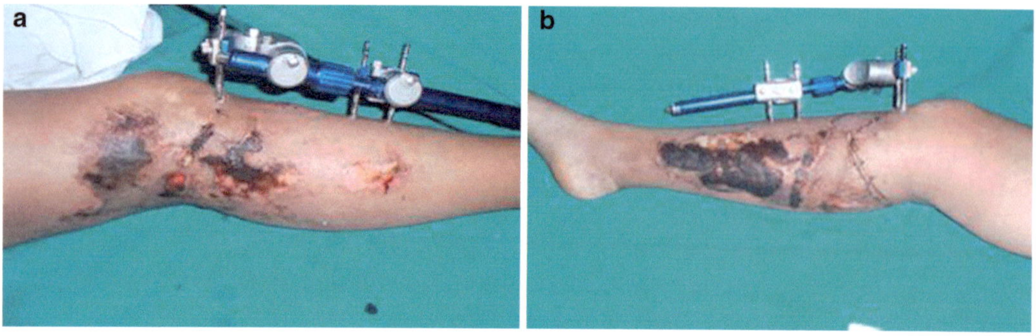

Fig. 2.12 Skin necrosis after Schatzker V fracture treated with external fixator: lateral view (**a**); medial view (**b**)

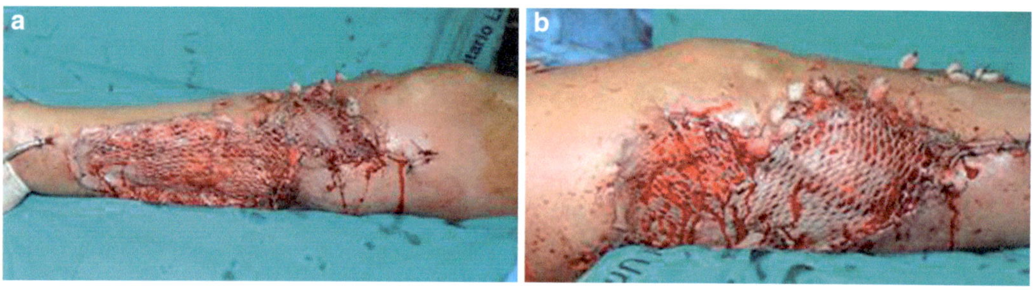

Fig. 2.13 The same case as in (Fig. 2.12). Débridement and coverage can be seen: medial view (**a**); lateral view (**b**)

2.5 Complications

As joint fractures, tibial plateau fractures can develop complications, some of them devastating. Complications can be divided into early, due to organic failures, and late, due to mechanical problems.

2.5.1 Early Complications

Skin Necrosis

Due to soft tissues damage, especially in complex fractures (Schatzker V and VI), the cutaneous circulation may be disrupted. Accordingly, skin necrosis can occur (Fig. 2.12).

Treatment of skin necrosis is wide débridement and then, skin coverage with autologous graft (Fig. 2.13).

Compartment Syndrome

It is a terrible complication that can lead to severe damage and even limb amputation. It is relatively common, appearing in 14.5 % of all cases [22] (Fig. 2.14). Its prevalence increases to 18 % in type VI fractures and to 53 % in type IV fractures [23]. However, it may go unnoticed especially if we do not think of it, in patients who have undergone high doses of analgesics or patients in coma. Measuring the pressure of the compartments can be useful for diagnosis but the clinical scene is prevalent. The management must be urgently by fascietomies of the four-leg compartments (Fig. 2.15).

Infection

Damage in the soft tissues around the fracture or inappropriate surgical approaches or both influence poor wound progress ending in deep infection [24].

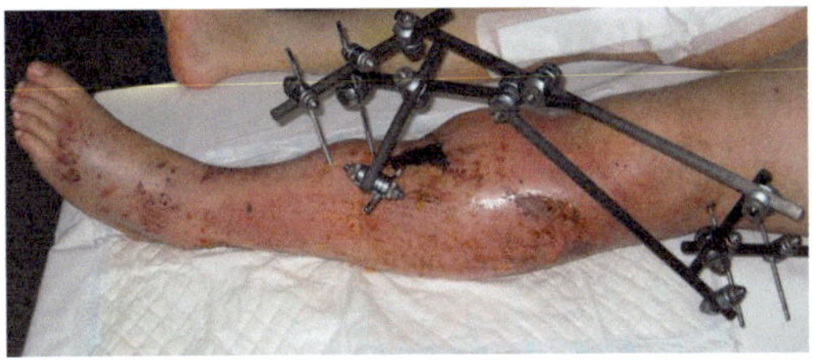

Fig. 2.14 Schatzker VI fracture treated by external fixator. It was complicated by a compartment syndrome

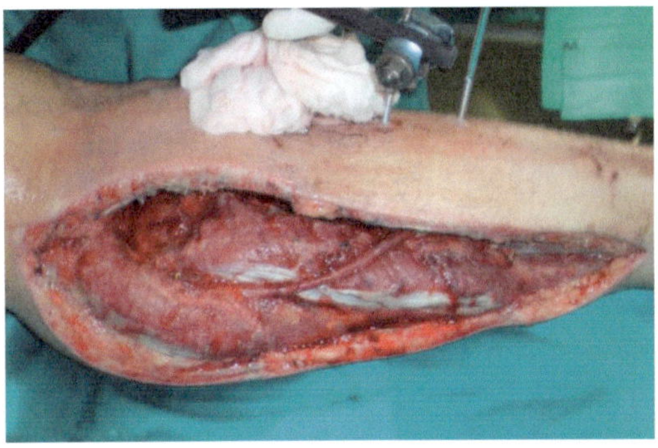

Fig. 2.15 Management of compartment syndrome by wide fasciotomy

If that occurs, surgical management is mandatory. Wound débridement, removing devitalized soft tissue, necrotic bone and irrigate thoroughly with antiseptic solution. Stable implants improving stability should not be removed. If a primary close cannot be done, a plastic coverage is indicated either by a pedicle flap or free flap. Intravenous antibiotic treatment is prescribed in each case depending on the antibiogram. The duration is 3–6 weeks (Fig. 2.16).

2.5.2 Late Complications

Nonunion

Nonunion in tibial plateau fractures is rare. It is more frequent in type VI fractures in the metaphyseal-diaphyseal junction as a result of mechanical instability, infection, or both [25]. Treatment is individualized. With no infection the treatment will consist of bone graft from iliac crest and stable osteosynthesis. But if infection is present, the treatment is done in two steps. First, débridement and washing is done followed by filling with cement with antibiotic and stabilizing with external fixator. Between 6 and 12 weeks later both external fixator and cement are removed. Then we bring bone graft and do an internal stable osteosynthesis.

Posttraumatic Osteoarthritis

Its frequency is high in these kinds of fractures (Fig. 2.17). It can get 30–40 % between the fifth and the tenth years [26, 27].Factors triggering posttraumatic osteoarthritis in the knee joint are three: joint incongruence, ligament injury with instability, and mechanical axis deviation. Treatment decision is conditioned by the patient age and location and severity of the osteoarthritis. In young patients with little affectation of one compartment and mechanical axis deviation, a corrective osteotomy can be indicated. By contrast, in elderly patients and/or severe affectation of two or three compartments, total knee replacement is indicated.

2.6 Conclusions

Tibial plateau fractures affect a large bearing joint. There is a bimodal distribution; they can affect young people after high-energy injury or can affect the elderly after low-energy injury on osteoporotic bone. Often accompanied by soft tissue injuries (types V and VI), they are sometimes complicated with neurologic or vascular damage (type IV). The goals of treatment are to restore the joint surface, provide stability, and get an anatomical load axis. Therefore, the treatment consists of anatomical reduction and stable fixation. However, the time of surgery is given by the soft tissue state. Early definitive surgery may be done when the soft tissues are well. Otherwise, a sequential management is preferred. The recommended surgical approaches are: anterolateral and posteromedial. Both

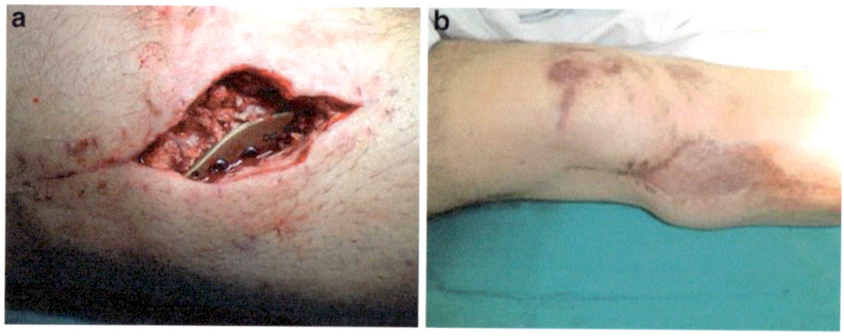

Fig. 2.16 Deep infection with hardware exposure (**a**); view after soft-tissue coverage (**b**)

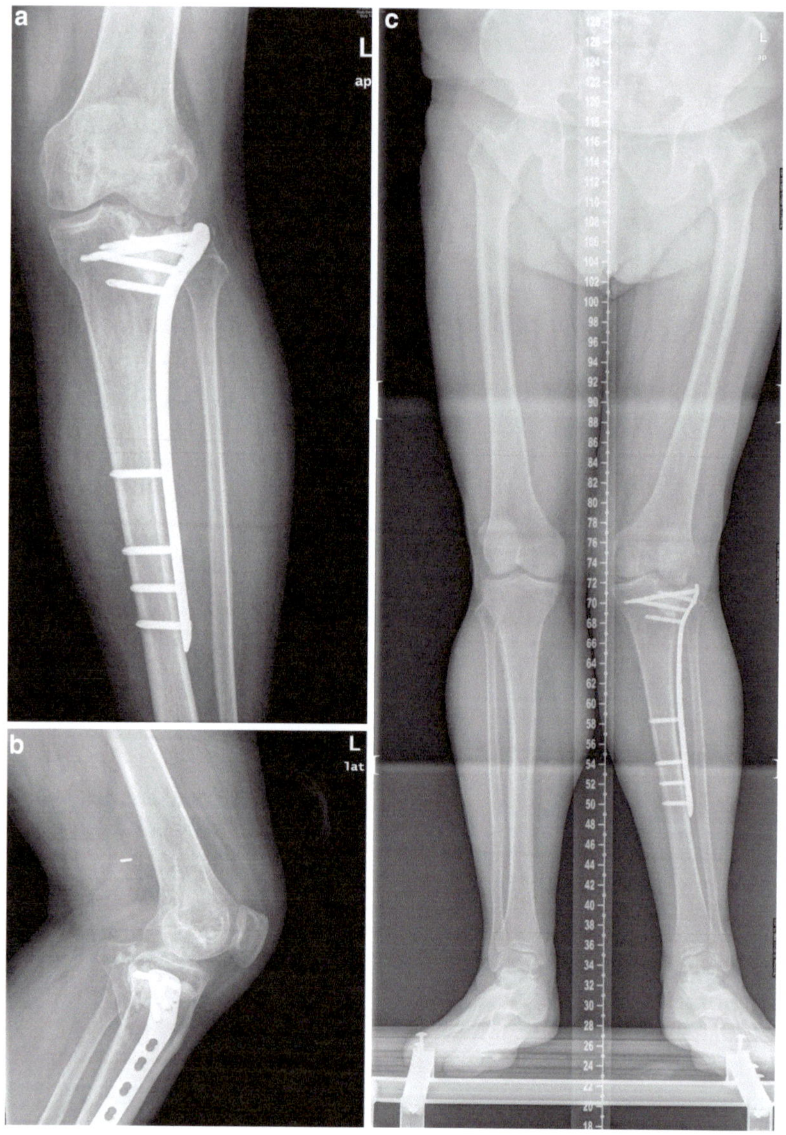

Fig. 2.17 Posttraumatic osteoarthritis after tibial plateau fracture: AP view (**a**); lateral view (**b**); AP standing radiographs (**c**)

should be done carefully in order to reduce the soft tissue injury and avoid further complications. Type I fractures can be managed by minimal invasive methods checking reduction by arthroscopic view and fixing the fracture by percutaneous cannulated screws. Type II and III fractures must be reduced by anterolateral approach; the articular fragment sunk has to be replaced and the remaining cavity has to be refilled with bone graft; finally, stabilization with plate must be done. Type IV fractures must be managed through posteromedial approach and fixed by medial osteosynthesis plate. Type V and VI fractures should be managed through two approaches and fixed with two plates, both lateral and medial ones. However, this kind of treatment could damage the soft tissues, thus in case of great soft tissue injury we can use the hybrid external fixation as an alternative treatment. Early complications, such as infection are frequent and the treatment consists of wide débridement and soft-tissue coverage. However, the most dangerous complication is the compartment syndrome. The best treatment is prevention so we should always remember it; if clinical signs of it exist, we must do four compartment fascietomies immediately.

References

1. Hohl M, Part I (1991) Fractures of the proximal tibia and fibula. In: Rockwood C, Green D, Bucholz R (eds) Fractures in adults, 3rd edn. JB Lippincott, Philadelphia, pp 1725–1761
2. Bennet WF, Browner B (1994) Tibial plateau fractures: a study of associated soft-tissue injuries. J Orthop Trauma 1994:183–188
3. Honkonen SE (1994) Indications for surgical treatment of tibial condyle fractures. Clin Orthop Relat Res May 302:199–205
4. Chan PS, Klimkiewicz JJ, Luchetti WT et al (1997) Impact of CT scan on treatment plan and fracture classification of tibial plateau fractures. J Orthop Trauma 11:484–489
5. Kode L, Lieberman JM, Motta AO et al (1994) Evaluation of tibial plateau fractures: efficacy of MR imaging compared with CT. Am J Roentgenol 163:141–147
6. Schatzker J (1987) Fractures of the tibial plateau. In: Schatzker J, Tile M (eds) Rationale of operative fracture care. Springer, New-York, p 279
7. Schatzker J (1993) Tibial plateau fractures. In: Bawner BD, Jupiter JB, Levine AM et al (eds) Skeletal Trauma. WB Saunders, Philadelphia, p 1745
8. Mitchell N, Shepard N (1980) Healing of articular cartilage in intraarticular fractures in rabbits. J Bone Joint Surg Am 62:628–634
9. Brown TD, Anderson DD, Nepola JV et al (1988) Contact stress aberrations following imprecise reduction of simple tibial plateau fracture. J Orthop Res 6:851–862
10. Tcherne H, Lobenhoffer P (1993) Tibial plateau fractures: management and expected results. Clin Orthop Relat Res 292:87–100
11. Watson JT, Coufal C (1998) Treatment of complex lateral plateau fractures using Ilizarov techniques. Clin Orthop Relat Res 353:97–106
12. Benirschke SK, Agnew SG, Mayo KA et al (1992) Inmediate external fixation of open complex tibial plateau fractures: treatment by a standard protocol. J Orthop Trauma 6:78–86
13. Waddell JP, Johnston DW, Neidre A (1981) Fractures of the tibial plateau: a review of 95 patients and comparison of treatment methods. J Trauma 21:376–381
14. Harper MC, Henstorf JE, Vessely MB (1995) Closed reductions and percutaneous stabilization of tibial plateau fractures. Orthopaedics 18:623–626
15. ItokazuM Matsunaga T, Ishii M et al (1996) Use of arthroscopy and interporous hydroxyapatite as a bone graft substitute in tibial plateau fractures: hydroxyapatite grafts. Arch Orthop TraumaSug 115:45–56
16. Itokazu M, Matsunaga T (1993) Arthroscopic restoration of depressed tibial plateau fractures using bone and hydroxyapatite grafts. Arthroscopy 9:103–108
17. Weiner LS, Kelley M, Yang E et al (1995) The use of combination internal fixation and hybrid external fixation in severe proximal tibial fractures. J Orthop Trauma 9:244–250
18. Marsh JL, Smith ST, Do TT (1995) External fixation and limited internal fixation for complex fractures of the tibial plateau. J Bone Joint Surg Am 77:661–673
19. Mikulak SA, Gold SM, Zinar DM (1998) Small wire external fixation of high energytibial plateau fractures. Clin Orthop Relat Res 356:230–238
20. Yong MJ, Barrack RL (1994) Complications of internal fixation of tibial plateau fractures. Orthop Rev 23:149–154
21. Segal D, Mallik AR, Wetzler MJ (1993) Early weight bearing of lateral tibial plateau fractures. Clin Orthop Relat Res 294:232–237
22. Barei DP, Nork SE, Mills WJ (2004) Complications associated with internal fixation of high-energy bicondylar tibial plateau fractures utilizing a two-incision technique. J Orthop Trauma 18:649–657
23. Stark EJ, Stucken C, Trainer G (2009) Compartment syndrome in Schatzker type VI plateau fractures and medial condylar fracture-dislocations treated with temporary external fixation. J Orthop Trauma 23:502–506

24. Mallik AR, Covall DJ, Whitelaw GP (1992) Internal versus external fixation of bicondylar tibial plateau fractures. Orthop Rev 21:1433–1436
25. Buckle R, Blake R, Watson JT et al (1993) Treatment of complex tibial plateau fractures with the Ilizarov external fixator. J Orthop Trauma 7:167
26. Honkonen SE (1995) Degenerative arthritis after tibial plateau fractures. J Orthop Trauma 9:273–277
27. Rademakers MV, Kerkhoffs GM, Sierevelt IN (2007) Operative treatment of 109 tibial plateau fractures: 5–27 year follow-up results. J Orthop Trauma 21:5–10

Patellar Fractures

3

Juan Sebastián Ruiz-Pérez, Ángel Martínez-Lloreda and E. Carlos Rodríguez-Merchán

3.1 Introduction

Patellar fractures account for approximately 0.5–1.5 % of all types of bone fractures [1]. The goal of treatment is restoring functional integrity of the extensor mechanism of the knee. Currently, the most widely accepted surgical technique for transverse patella fractures is open reduction and internal fixation with a modified AO tension band [2, 3]. This principle converts the tension forces acting on the anterior surface into compression forces at the articular surface. This technique can substantially improve results because of its reliable fixation and allowance of early joint motion. However, symptoms and complications related to this technique are not uncommon, such as wire breakage, migration and prominent hardware in the knee, loss of reduction, migration of fracture fragments, and soft-tissue irritation. This remains a challenge for the orthopedic surgeon leading to the development of therapeutic alternatives and design of new implants. The purpose of this chapter is to revise current knowledge on patellar fractures.

3.2 Anatomy and Biomechanics

The patella, the largest human sesamoid bone, lies within and is an important functional component of the knee extensor mechanism, along with two other elements such as the quadriceps tendon and patellar tendon. The patellar retinaculum also contributes to this function and is composed of fibers of the tensor fascia lata and fascia of both vast, lateral, and medial hugging the patella along its range of movement. Its subcutaneous location, makes it likely to appear in the context of open fractures after direct trauma.

The posterior view is covered by the thickest cartilage of human body. Patella presents two facet joints, lateral and medial, separated by a vertical septum and originates from a single nucleus of ossification. However, in 2–3 % of the population may appear secondary ossification nucleus between 8 and 12 years of age and remain as independent fragment. The anomaly is bilateral is approximately 50 % of individuals. Green classified bipartite patella in three groups based on the position of the accessory center: type I, inferior pole; type II, lateral margin; and type III, superolateral pole (75 % of the cases) [4]. Bipartite patella should not be confused with fracture.

The blood supply is provided by anastomotic ring originating from the geniculate arteries which penetrate in the thickness of the anterior

J. S. Ruiz-Pérez (✉) · Á. Martínez-Lloreda ·
E. C. Rodríguez-Merchán
Department of Orthopaedic Surgery, "La Paz" University Hospital-IdiPaz, Paseo de la Castellana 261, 28046, Madrid, Madrid, Spain
e-mail: juanseruizperez@hotmail.com

Á. Martínez-Lloreda
e-mail: angelmlloreda@gmail.com

E. C. Rodríguez-Merchán
e-mail: ecrmerchan@gmx.es

E. C. Rodríguez-Merchán (ed.), *Traumatic Injuries of the Knee*,
DOI: 10.1007/978-88-470-5298-7_3, © Springer-Verlag Italia 2013

surface and the infrapatellar fat. In its upper portion, the anastomotic circuit, runs above the quadriceps tendon, while in the lower area is located posterior to the patellar tendon. This is the reason why the circumferential dissection should be avoided. Although the incidence of osteonecrosis secondary to fracture has been reported to be as high as 25 %, clinical outcomes were not affected.

Its main function is to allow active extension of the joint and keep the body upright against gravity. Patella acts as a pulley increasing the moment arm of the quadriceps by up to 30 % [5]. Loading patterns about the patella are complex. The quadriceps loads the patella in tension. However, with knee flexion, posterior surface of quadriceps tendon also comes into contact with the trochlea; when this occurs, compressive forces on the patellofemoral articulation are diminished owing to division of the load bearing between patellofemoral joint and the tendon of quadriceps mechanism.

Activities such as climbing stairs can generate compressive forces on the patellofemoral joint greater than seven times the body weight bearing the anterior patellar surface at values close to fracture risk.

3.3 Mechanism of Injury

Patella fractures may occur as a result of direct or indirect trauma. A direct force consists of a direct blow to the anterior knee from a fall or dashboard injury resulting in a comminuted or stellate fracture pattern. Mostly of these fractures are non-displaced, although cartilage damage must be taken into account. Moreover, the patella may suffer an indirect force when extensor mechanism of the knee exceeds the strength of the bone resulting in transverse fracture or avulsion of the inferior pole. The force often continues beyond the patella, extending through the retinaculum causing loss of active knee extension. Less common causes correspond to insufficiency fractures after obtaining bone grafting for reconstruction of anterior cruciate ligament (ACL) injuries and knee arthroplasty.

3.4 Clinical Presentation and Physical Examination

History of a direct blow to the knee or eccentric loading should raise suspicion for patellar fracture or other extensor mechanism injury. Orthopedic surgeons must be aware of the presence of associated injuries in the context of high-energy trauma against the dashboard as hip, acetabulum, distal femur fractures, and knee dislocations.

The knee examination begins with inspection of the soft-tissue envelope. At first sight it is often found swelling, erosion, ecchymosis, and a gap on the patellar surface with limitations in knee active extension. Palpation reveals hemarthrosis, pain with palpation, and a palpable defect. It is essential to ensure that any wound in this area does not communicate with the joint or fracture; load test performed with intraarticular injection of saline solution may be helpful.

3.5 Radiographic Evaluation

Standard AP and lateral radiographs of the knee should be obtained. Lateral radiographs are useful in assessing displacement and articular congruity in patients with transverse fractures. Anteroposterior view may be not helpful because of the superimposition of the patella with the femoral condyles and axial view is only recommendable for vertical fractures. Any other radiological tests (CT, MRI) are rarely indicated except in the case of suspected joint damage as osteochondral injury (Fig. 3.1).

3.6 Classification

Patellar fractures are classified descriptively according to fracture pattern [6]. The most common types are transverse not-comminuted, multifragmentary, or avulsion fractures Transverse fractures appear in young patients with good bone quality. Avulsion fractures of the upper or lower pole are functionally equivalent to disruptions of union tendon-bone of patellar

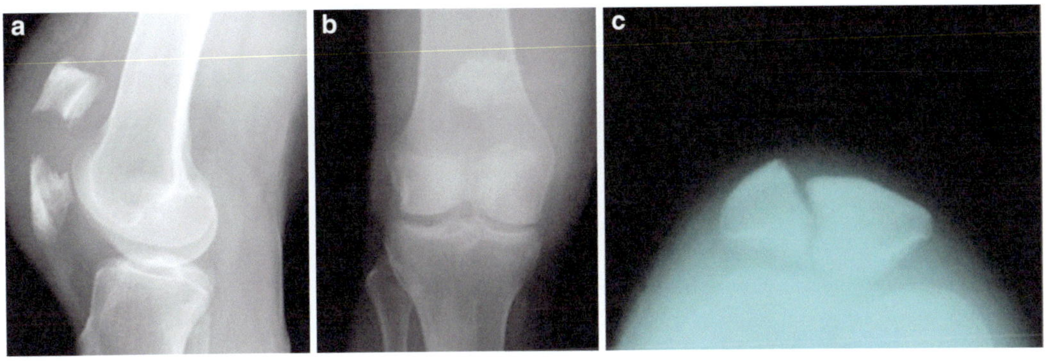

Fig. 3.1 Standard AP (**a**) and lateral (**b**) views of a transverse patellar fracture. (**c**) Skyline view of a vertical patellar fracture

or quadriceps tendon. Attending to displacement, patellar fractures may be classified as non-displaced or displaced (step-off > 2–3 mm and fracture gap > 1–4 mm). Classification often predicts treatment. The Orthopaedic Trauma Association (OTA/AO) classification is based on degree of articular involvement and number of fracture fragments [6].

3.7 Management

The goal of treatment must be to achieve the anatomical reduction of both the fracture and the articular surface in addition to stable fixation of the fracture, which allows early rehabilitation of the knee. Every effort should be made to preserve as much patellar bone as possible.

3.7.1 Conservative Treatment

In fractures with mínimum articular displacement (step-off and/or fracture displacement – < 2–3 mm and <1–4 mm, respectively) and intact extensor mechanism may be an attempt of nonsurgical treatment. It is recommended a weight-bearing period with the knee in full extension immobilized with a Böhler cylindrical plaster or locked brace during 4–6 weeks. Isometric quadriceps exercise and straight leg raises are begun when pain has subsided. Afterwards, progressive passive and active motion is allowed.

Boström [7] used plaster immobilization for a mean duration of 4 weeks to manage patellar fractures with an intact extensor mechanism. Good or excellent outcomes were reported in 99 % of fractures at a mean 9-year follow-up.

Braun et al. reported 40 cases with less than 1 mm of displacement treated conservatively with 80 % of the patients without pain and 90 % had full range of motion at a mean 30.5 months after injury [8].

Pritchet [9] presented 18 patients with displaced fractures >1 cm in cases whose activities were limited by chronic illness. Only three patients had limitations on their basic daily activities considering this therapy as definitive treatment in the patient with significant medical comorbidities. No patient had severe pain, but all patients had extensor lag of ≥20°.

3.7.2 Surgical Treatment

The main indication for surgical treatment is restoring an incompetent extensor mechanism of the knee. Typically other common indications may be articular damage, fracture separation >1–4 mm and step-off >2–3 mm, intra-articular loose bodies from osteochondral injuries. The goal of the therapy should be anatomical reduction of both the fracture and the articular surface in addition to the stable fixation.

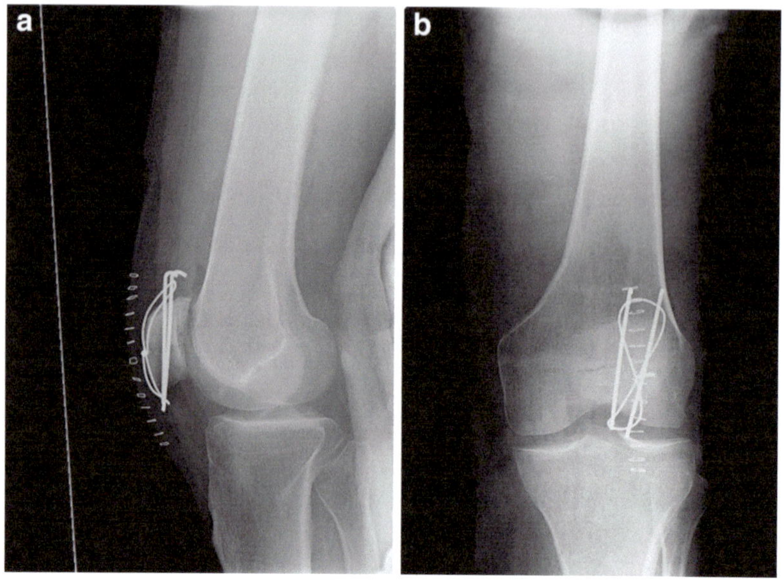

Fig. 3.2 Postoperative radiograph of Modified Tension Band Wiring-8 figure. (**a**) AP view. (**b**) Lateral radiograph

Tension-Band Wiring

Currently, the most widely accepted surgical technique for transverse patella fractures is open reduction and internal fixation with a modified AO tension band. This technique was introduced in the 1950s. Several studies [2] demonstrated the superiority of this technique compared with other fixation methods. Since then, multiple variations on the technique have been described. However, postoperative complications are common with this method, including loss of motion, malunion, and symptomatic hardware [10].

The preferred approach to these fractures should be a longitudinal midline incision over the patella avoiding circumferential dissection of subcutaneous and fascia tissue. Nevertheless for transverse fractures two flaps, lateral and medial, may allow access to retinacular tears. Several different incisions have been described. Gardner et al. [11] advocated lateral parapatellar arthrotomy for direct visual reduction of comminuted fractures allowing for direct application of instrumentation to the bony surfaces, without soft-tissue interposition. Transverse approaches should not be used.

Currently, tension-band wiring remains the most commonly used technique for the management of patellar fracture. This technique converts the anterior tension forces of the extensor mechanism and knee flexion into compression forces at the articular surface. Several variations of this technique have been described (standard, modified tension-band and an eight-figure over the patellar surface) (Fig. 3.2).

Modified tension-band wiring (MTBW) in a figure of-eight pattern looped over the anterior patella is the most widely accepted method of fixation for transverse fractures. Standard wiring [12] and eight-figure configuration permitted less separation of fracture fragments than either circumferential wiring or standard tension-band wiring. This is one of the reasons that the standard technique has been abandoned in favor of the newest MTBW (Fig. 3.3).

Lefaivre et al. [12] reported a case series of 31 patients using a modified tension band technique for patella fractures with four K wires capturing the figure of eight wire. Four cases had hardware removed for irritation despite satisfactory post-operative radiographic results and one patient had a nonunion without failure of hardware, and was revised to compression screws at 7 months post-operative.

Fortis et al. [13] described in a cadaveric model a new design for a MTBW demonstrating increase compressive strain in a transverse

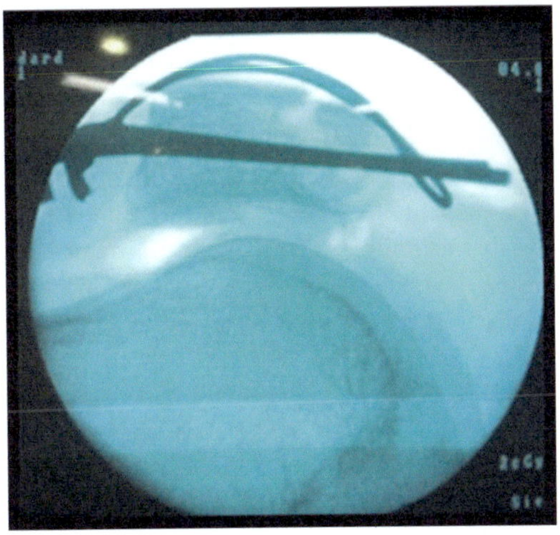

Fig. 3.3 Intraoperative view of a patellar fracture after reduction and internal fixation

fracture improved by an additional circular wire. Lotke and Ecker wiring system [14], a longitudinal anterior band which a wire is pulled and looped over the surface of the patella, seems insufficient in patients that need to recover full activity as soon as possible. John et al. [15] developed a wooden model of a transversely fractured patella to compare different fixation constructs. Placement of the figure of eight in a horizontal orientation with two wire twists at the corner improved interfragmentary compression by 63 % and permanent fracture displacement after cyclic loading was 67 % lower with horizontal figure of eight constructs.

Rathi et al. [16] evaluated outcomes of percutaneous tension band wiring for transverse fractures of the patella in 23 patients. The objective score was excellent in 20 patients and good in three. All patients had radiological union at week eight. Three patients encountered hardware problems necessitating implant removal.

Screws Fixation and Tension-Band

Screws offer better biomechanical performance than do longitudinal K-wires in the MTBW construct. Several authors have focus into this line in cases with a good bone stock [17, 18]. It is rather difficult to place the tension-band wires around the tips and heads of screws. Berg [18] reported a case series of ten patients. Subjective and functional results using Hospital for Special Surgery Knee Scores were comparable to previously published reports, with 70 percent achieving an excellent or good outcome. LeBrun et al. [19] presented 40 patients with patellar fractures at mean follow-up of 6.5 years treated with standard tension band with Kirschner wires, tension band through 2 cannulated screws, longitudinal anterior banding with cerclage, or partial patellectomy. Removal of symptomatic fixation was required in 52 % of the patients whereas 38 % of those with retained fixation self- reported implant-related pain at least some of the time. A restricted range of flexion/extension of >5° was noted in 38 % and 15 % of the cases, respectively. Tian et al. [20] conducted a retrospective comparison between modified tensión band and titanium cable-cannulated technique in 101 patients. This second group showed superior results in fracture reduction, reduced healing time, and better Iowa score considering as an alternative method for treatment of transverse patellar fractures.

3.7.3 Alternative Treatments

Although this management is historically accepted it has been necessary investigate new designs and alternatives to wire constructs. Braided polyester sutures are the most extensively researched alternative. McGreal et al. [21] described sixteen cadaveric patellae which were fractured and repaired by modified tension band fixation (stainless Steel wire vs braided polyester). Polyester was 75.0 % as strong as wire concluding that polyester is an acceptable alternative to wire in tension band fixation. Gosal et al. [22] compared patellar fractures managed with MTBW with stainless steel wire to those cases managed with two braided polyester sutures (No. 5 Ethibond). Therefore, the relative risk of reoperation in the metal group is six times that in the non-absorbable polyester group (38 % vs 6 %) and risk of infection in the metal group is also higher. According to these authors non absorbable polyester appears to compare favourably with the use of metallic wire to fix patellar fractures. Qi et al. [23] in the attempt to find new materials involving minor local complications in the surgical área presented fifteen patients with displaced transverse or comminuted patella who were treated using bioabsorbable cannulated lag screws and braided polyester suture tension bands. The mean knee joint range of motion was from 0 to 134 and the mean VAS score was 0.7 at the time of bone union. No postoperative complications, such as infection, dislocation or breakage of the implants, were observed.

Yang et al. [24] described a new surgical technique particularly useful in comminuted fractures when patellar excision would otherwise be considered. This author trialed titanium cable cerclage in 21 patients followed up for a mean period of 24 months. The mean score at the final follow-up was 27 points (25–30). It means the functional results were excellent in 81 %, and good in 19 % of the cases. There was no complication except breakage of one cable at the sixth week after the operation.

Another interesting study [25] showed a 2.7 mm fixed-angle plate designed for the treatment of patella fractures. It was tested biomechanically against other fixation methods like modified anterior tension wiring or cannulated lag screws with anterior tension wiring. Those patellae stabilized with fixed-angle plates showed no significant fracture gap widening after completion of 100 cycles. They summarize that in cyclic biomechanical testing on human cadaver knees the bilateral fixed-angle plate proved to be a rigid, stable, and sustainable fixation device for transverse patella fractures.

Minimally Invasive Techniques

Less invasive techniques have been developed in order to minimize soft-tissue injuries. Luna-Pizarro et al. [26] compared a new percutaneous patellar osteosynthesis system technique with open surgery for patella fractures in 53 patients. This percutaneous technique was associated with shorter surgical time, less pain, better mobility angles, higher functional score up to 2 years, and a lower incidence of complications. A total of 31 patients with displaced transverse fractures of the patella were operatively treated by a Cable Pin System [27] with a minimally invasive technique. The average Bostman score was 29.1 at 1 year after surgery, and an evaluation of "excellent" was observed in 30 patients at the final follow-up visit.

Arthroscopic therapies [28] have also been described. However, authors of these articles stress careful selection of patients suitable for these techniques and acknowledge the inability to address tears of other structures like the retinaculum.

Open Patellar Fractures

These fractures represent 6–9 % of total patellar fractures [29]. They are observed in the context of high energy trauma as a result of motor vehicle collisions, with nearly 70 % accompanied by other injuries. Management of these fractures involves balancing a need for soft tissue healing versus the benefit of early movement enabled by stable fixation. Anand et al. [29] observed that open fractures were associated with a poorer functional outcome and more complications. In contrast to this study Catalano et al. [30] reported 79 open fractures treated with irrigation and débridement, open reduction, internal fixation, and reconstruction of the extensor mechanism. At an average of 36 months, good to excellent knee scores were observed in 17 of 22 patients and average range of motion for all groups was 112°. They conclude that all attempts for preservation of bone substance and precise reconstruction of the extensor should be attempted, reserving total patellectomy as a salvage procedure. Wardak et al. [31] proposed an alternative treatment with a system based on the Ilizarov method. 84 patients (26 open fractures, cases with a poor soft tissue envelope, salvage situations) at an average follow-up of 4 years were treated with the technique of compressive external fixation (CEF), a device based on an external tensioned wire construct. All of the fractures attained union. The device was removed in the office at 6 weeks. Insall knee score was 97 points and minor complications (wire irritation) presented in 11 % of patients. We recommend urgent and meticulous débridement, irrigation, and definitive fixation. All attempts are made to preserve bone; patellectomy is reserved for selected cases of substantial bone loss. Skin grafting or flap coverage may be useful in cases with extensive soft-tissue damage. It will help to minimize the risk of infection and promote fracture healing.

Partial Patellectomy and Inferior Pole Fracture

Inferior pole fractures of the patella, or those multifragmentary close to inferior pole may be treated with partial patellectomy and patellar tendon advancement. Normally three holes are made with a drill through the upper pole in longitudinal direction. Then several nonabsorbable braided sutures are placed as locking points crossing patellar tendon and they are passed through those holes and knotted in the upper pole. Sometimes It is not necessary to remove small comminuted fragments from the inferior pole of the patella and it may help fracture healing. Cerclage reinforcement with a strong suture can be useful. Saltzman et al. [32] described partial patellectomy in 40 patients with transverse or inferior pole fractures of the patella. Excellent and good results were reported in 78 % of the cases and mean quadriceps strength was found to be 85 % that of the contralateral knee. Yang and Byun [33] evaluated the clinical effectiveness of the separate vertical wiring technique in acute comminuted fractures of the inferior pole of the patella getting a 100 % union rate. A basket plate osteosynthesis was compared with partial patellectomy in a study [34] for an average of 5.3 years. Significant differences between the groups were noted with regard to knee pain, swallowing, level activity, compression pain, range of motion, muscular atrophy, muscular strength, and final patellofemoral score in favor of the base plate group with excellent or good results in 90.1 % patients.

Total Patellectomy

Indications for total patellectomy have diminished. Total patellectomy may result in a >49 % reduction in quadriceps strength so every attempt should be made to retain bone stock. This technique should only be performed in extreme cases such infection, open fractures, tumors, patellofemoral arthritis, or previous failed fixation. Advancing the vastus medialis obliquus muscle may increase strength and outcomes of total patellectomy.

3.8 Rehabilitation

No data exist on outcomes for specific postoperative protocols, but in our experience we strongly recommend early rehabilitation protocol after and initial period of non weight-bearing with a circular cast in full extension for the first 2 weeks. Then isometric quadriceps exercises are allowed with partial weight-bearing assisted with crutches for the next 4–6 weeks. At this moment passive and active motion of the knee is started. Return to intense physical activity is usually delayed until the third postoperative month. If tenuous internal fixation or partial patellectomy is performed standard in mobilization should be maintained until 6 weeks.

3.9 Complications

Most frequent complication is symptomatic hardware (0–60 %) [14, 18, 19]. Smith et al. [10] reported a hardware failure rate of 8–22 %. Lose of reduction and wire migration are one of the most feared complications. Miller et al. [35] performed a retrospective study of 173 patients with patellar fractures in order to identify predictors of surgical treatment failure. It was defined as hardware breakage, nonunion, or displacement of fragments from their initial reduced position. Twelve factors were examined independently. Both older patient age and use of K-wires, with or without tension-band wires), were found to be significant predictors of failure.

Table 3.1 Complications of surgical treatment of patellar fractures

Infection	11 %
Fixation failure	22 %
Symptomatic hardware	20–60 %
Non-union	2.7–12.5 %

Use of K-wires with or without tension-band wires correlated with higher failure rates, compared with the use of screws (Table 3.1).

The incidence of non-union or delayed union of patellar fractures ranges from 2.7 to 12.5 % [36]. Several studies suggest that certain factors such as open fractures, improper immobilization, and the initial fracture configuration may raise orthopedic surgeon vigilance. Patients with low functional demand should be managed with non-operative treatment instead of those who perform heavy physical work that usually require open reduction and internal fixation. Tension band wiring is the treatment of choice for a reconstructive procedure. Partial or total patellectomy is also an option where satisfactory internal fixation cannot be achieved [37].

Knee stiffness is another possible shortcoming. Many authors advocate internal fixation to allow early motion. Length of immobilization seems to be related with stiffness but it is not clear. Total and partial patellectomy may cause substantial knee extensor weakness.

Patellar fracture has been associated with increased rates of patellofemoral osteoarthritis (16–53 %) [7, 32] although the contribution of the injury force compared with the quality of reduction remains unclear.

3.10 Conclusions

Patellar fractures are frequently associated with extensor weakness, stiffness, and patellofemoral osteoarthritis. Fracture displacement (step off >2–3 mm and gap >1–4 mm) and integrity of extensor mechanism of the knee determine definitive treatment. Currently, tension-band wiring remains the most commonly used technique for the management of patellar fracture. However, symptoms and complications related to this technique have been described widely in classic literature. Cannulated screws tension-band, instead typical stainless steel wires, and early ROM are associated with the best outcomes. The development of new implants may improve future functional results. Total patellectomy should only be considered in extreme cases. Every effort should be made to preserve patellar bone stock.

References

1. Weber MJ, Janecki CJ, McLeod P, Nelson CL, Thompson JA (1980) Efficacy of various forms of fixation of transverse fractures of the patella. J Bone Joint Surg Am 62:215–220
2. Hung LK, Chan KM, Chow YN, Leung PC (1985) Fractured patella: operative treatment using the tension band principle. Injury 16:343–347
3. Nummi J (1971) Operative treatment of patellar fractures. Acta Orthop Scand 42:437–438
4. Green WT Jr (1975) Painful bipartite patella: a report of three cases. Clin Orthop Relat Res 110:197–200
5. Kaufer H (1971) Mechanical function of the patella. J Bone Joint Surg Am 53:1551–1560
6. Marsh JL, Slongo TF, Agel J, Broderick JS, Creevey W, DeCoster TA, Prokuski L, Sirkin MS, Ziran B, Henley B, Audigé L (2007) Fracture and dislocation classification compendium-2007: Orthopaedic Trauma Association classification, database and outcomes committee. J Orthop Trauma 21(10 Suppl):S1–S133
7. Boström A (1972) Fracture of the patella: a study of 422 patellar fractures. Acta Orthop Scand Suppl 143:1–80
8. Braun W, Wiedemann M, Rüter A, Kundel K, Kolbinger S (1993) Indications and results of nonoperative treatment of patellar fractures. Clin Orthop Relat Res 289:197–201
9. Pritchett JW (1997) Nonoperative treatment of widely displaced patella fractures. Am J Knee Surg 10:145–147
10. Smith ST, Cramer KE, Karges DE, Watson JT, Moed BR (1997) Early complications in the operative treatment of patella fractures. J Orthop Trauma 11:183–187
11. Gardner MJ, Griffith MH, Lawrence BD, Lorich DG (2005) Complete exposure of the articular surface for fixation of patellar fractures. J Orthop Trauma 19:118–123
12. Lefaivre KA, O'Brien PJ, Broekhuyse HM, Guy P, Blachut PA (2010) Modified tension band technique for patella fractures. Orthop Traumatol Surg Res 96:579–582

13. Fortis AP, Milis Z, Kostopoulos V et al (2002) Experimental investigation of the tension band in fractures of the patella. Injury 33:489–493
14. Lotke PA, Ecker ML (1981) Transverse fractures of the patella. Clin Orthop Relat Res 158:180–184
15. John J, Wagner WW, Kuiper JH (2007) Tension-band wiring of transverse fractures of patella: The effect of site of wire twists and orientation of stainless steel wire loop. A biomechanical investigation. Int Orthop 31:703–707
16. Rathi A, Swamy MK, Prasantha I, Consul A, Bansal A, Bahl V (2012) Percutaneous tension band wiring for patellar fractures. J Orthop Surg (Hong Kong) 20:166–169
17. Burvant JG, Thomas KA, Alexander R, Harris MB (1994) Evaluation of methods of internal fixation of transverse patella fractures: a biomechanical study. J Orthop Trauma 8:147–153
18. Berg EE (1997) Open reduction internal fixation of displaced transverse patella fractures with figure-eight wiring through parallel cannulated compression screws. J Orthop Trauma 11:573–576
19. LeBrun CT, Langford JR, Sagi HC (2012) Functional outcomes after operatively treated patella fractures. J Orthop Trauma 26:422–426
20. Tian Y, Zhou F, Ji H, Zhang Z (2011) Cannulated screw and cable are superior to modified tension band in the treatment of transverse patella fractures. Clin Orthop Relat Res 469:3429–3433
21. McGreal G, Reidy D, Joy A, Mahalingam K, Cashman WF (1999) The biomechanical evaluation of polyester as a tension band for the internal fixation of patellar fractures. J Med Eng Technol 23:53–56
22. Gosal HS, Singh P, Field RE (2001) Clinical experience of patellar fracture fixation using metal wire or non-absorbable polyester: a study of 37 cases. Injury 32:129–135
23. Qi L, Chang C, Xin T, Xing PF, Tianfu Y, Gang Z, Jian L (2011) Double fixation of displaced patella fractures using bio absorbable cannulated lag screws and braided polyester suture tension bands. Injury 42:1116–1120
24. Yang L, Yueping O, Wen Y (2010) Management of displaced comminuted patellar fracture with titanium cable cerclage. Knee 17:283–286
25. Thelen S, Schneppendahl J, Jopen E, Eichler C, Koebke J, Schönau E, Hakimi M, Windolf J, Wild M (2012) Biomechanical cadaver testing of a fixed angle plate in comparison to tension wiring and screw fixation in transverse patella fractures. Injury 43:1290–1295
26. Luna-Pizarro D, Amato D, Arellano F, Hernández A, López-Rojas P (2006) Comparison of a technique using a new percutaneous osteosynthesis device with conventional open surgery for displaced patella fractures in a randomized controlled trial. J Orthop Trauma 20:529–535
27. Mao N, Ni H, Ding W, Zhu X, Bai Y, Wang C, Zhao Y, Shi Z, Li M, Zhang Q (2012) Surgical treatment of transverse patella fractures by the cable pin system with animally invasive technique. J Trauma Acute Care Surg 72:1056–1061
28. El-Sayed AM, Ragab RK (2009) Arthroscopic-assisted reduction and stabilization of transverse fractures of the patella. Knee 16:54–57
29. Anand S, Hahnel JC, Giannoudis PV (2008) Open patellar fractures: high energy injuries with a poor outcome? Injury 39:480–484
30. Catalano JB, Iannacone WM, Marczyk S et al (1995) Open fractures of the patella: long-term functional outcome. J Trauma 39:439–444
31. Wardak MI, Siawash AR, Hayda R (2012) Fixation of patella fractures with a minimally invasive tensioned wire method: compressive external fixation. J Trauma Acute Care Surg 72:1393–1398
32. Saltzman CL, Goulet JA, McClellan RT, Schneider LA, Matthews LS (1990) Results of treatment of displaced patellar fractures by partial patellectomy. J Bone Joint Surg Am 72:1279–1285
33. Yang KH, Byun YS (2003) Separate vertical wiring for the fixation of comminuted fractures of the inferior pole of the patella. J Bone Joint Surg Br 85:1155–1160
34. Matejcić A, Puljiz Z, Elabjer E, Bekavac- Beslin M, Ledinsky M (2008) Multifragment fracture of the patellar apex: Basket plate osteosynthesis compared with partial patellectomy. Arch Orthop Trauma Surg 128:403–408
35. Miller MA, Liu W, Zurakowski D, Smith RM, Harris MB, Vrahas MS (2010) Factors predicting failure of patella fixation. J Trauma Acute Care Surg 72:1051–1055
36. Klassen JF, Trousdale RT (1997) Treatment of delayed and nonunion of the patella. J Orthop Trauma 11:188–194
37. Nathan ST, Fisher BE, Roberts CS, Giannoudis PV (2011) The management of nonunion and delayed union of patella fractures: a systematic review of the literature. Int Orthop 35:791–795

Patellar Dislocations and Osteochondral Fractures

4

Eduardo García-Rey

4.1 Introduction

Acute patellar dislocations are a common problem for the orthopaedic surgeon that can lead to recurrent instability and chronic anterior knee pain in young patients [1]. This is an important topic due to several reasons. The incidence is quite high particularly in teenagers and, although early management used to be conservative, surgical treatment may be necessary for many of them [2]. The rate of redislocation is also higher in younger patients and the associated pathological findings are very frequent (Fig. 4.1). When a patient presents this injury, the surgeon must carefully evaluate all conditions around the knee in order to offer the best solution.

4.2 Primary Dislocation of the Patella

A first-time patellar dislocation is usually very disabling for the patient who frequently reports "my knee has gone away"; the physician may observe a very painful and swelling knee after doing a sport (very often a team contact sport). Most of the times the patella has been reduced spontaneously before the adolescent arrives to the Emergency Department and makes the diagnoses difficult. Sometimes the patellar dislocation is well recognised and the reduction can be made gently. In other rare cases this is not possible and an open surgical intervention might be necessary due to a complete torn of the vastus medialis obliquus from the medial aspect of the patella.

The exploration of the knee must be very cautious, the hemarthroses is removed and ligament stability is checked, particularly when the dislocation has been reduced before the medical assistance. The medial retinaculum of the patella is very painful as well as the patient shows fear when trying to subluxated laterally.

Radiological examinations may recognise any bone or osteochondral lesions on all views (antero-posterior, lateral and true skyline view of the patella) (Fig. 4.2). In patients with previous contralateral patellar dislocation, the physician must check all abnormalities on the femoral trochlea as well as the type of patella according to Wiberg [3]. Then the surgeon must decide which is the best treatment for each patient.

Conservative treatment has been classically the initial management for these lesions. An adequate reduction, immobilization and an intensive rehabilitation program offer a good result for many patients. For a better understanding, it is mandatory to remember the pathology of the lesion. Medial retinaculum tissues are formed by the medial patellofemoral

E. García-Rey (✉)
Department of Orthopaedic Surgery, "La Paz" University Hospital-Idipaz,
Paseo de la Castellana 261, 28046, Madrid, Spain
e-mail: edugrey@yahoo.es

E. C. Rodríguez-Merchán (ed.), *Traumatic Injuries of the Knee*,
DOI: 10.1007/978-88-470-5298-7_4, © Springer-Verlag Italia 2013

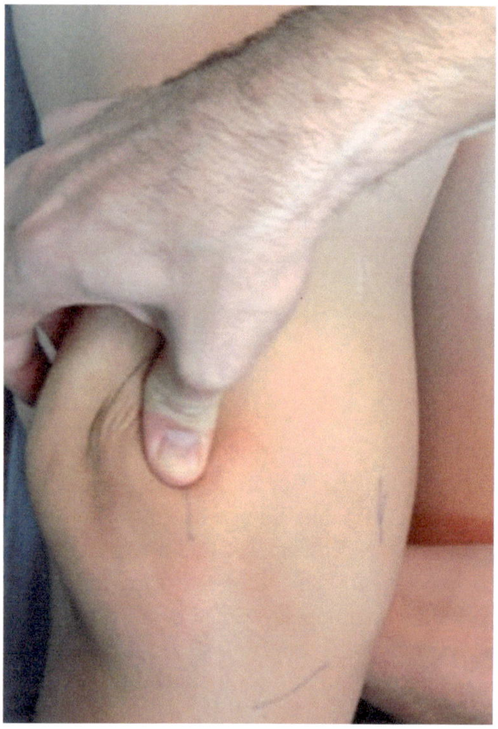

Fig. 4.1 Examination of the knee of a 14-year-old-female patient who suffered a second episode of patellar dislocation

ligament (MPFL), the superficial medial retinaculum and the medial patellotibial ligament (Fig. 4.1). Half of the total forces that are necessary to dislocate the patella are provided by the MPFL, this contribution is particularly high when the knee is extended [4]. It is also well known that vastus medialis muscle acts like a secondary stabiliser, and inefficient when is relaxed [5]. Waligora et al. described that MPFL does not always exits and runs between the medial femoral condyle and the superolateral corner of the patella, is usually very wide and has an extensive connection to the vastus medialis [6]. Nomura classified the pathology of this lesion as an avulsion-tear type, from the distal medial femoral attachment, or intrasubstantial-tear for acute dislocations [7].

The type of immobilization may vary from a bandage, posterior splint or a cast, as well as the time, from 3 to 6 weeks. The posterior splint during 6 weeks seems to allow an adequate immobilization to prevent redislocation without a high degree of stiffness; this is probably due to the patient who can start doing isometric exercises with his/her quadriceps muscle [8].

However, conservative treatment is not always successful as mentioned above. After the initial management of the lesion a complete medical history must be made. Previous episodes on the contralateral knee must alert the orthopaedic surgeon and look for anatomic abnormalities. Radiological images may show associated bone lesions such as fractures or osteochondral fragments. Thus, if these images are not enough to demonstrate any fracture and hemarthroses at present, a magnetic resonance imaging (MRI) must be prescribed. This tool allows describing any osteochondral abnormalities as well as other findings related to the trochlea, femoral condyle, cartilage status and other soft-tissue problems [9].

Management of lateral dislocation of the patella without associated bone lesions continues to be controversial so the orthopaedic surgeon must know the results of every type of treatment conservative or not. Table 4.1 tries to summarise this issue. Prospective comparative, particularly randomised, studies are the best way to review this topic. Nikku et al. in a long-term randomised study, observed similar results for both conservative and realigning the extensor mechanism and repairing the medial patellar ligament according to the individual pathoanatomy [10]. They emphasised the importance of female sex in the rate of redislocation more than the mode of treatment, as well as the clinical descriptions and differences between relocation-dislocation and "locked dislocation". Thus, other factors such as family history, contralateral lesion and loose bodies also determines clinical outcome for these patients. Christiansen et al. assessed the clinical outcome and redislocation rate of delayed primary repair of the medial patellofemoral ligament by use of an anchor and the conservative treatment of primary dislocation of the patella by use a brace; they did not observe any differences between groups but for a better patellar clinical result for the surgical treatment [11]. Sillanpää et al. observed a better

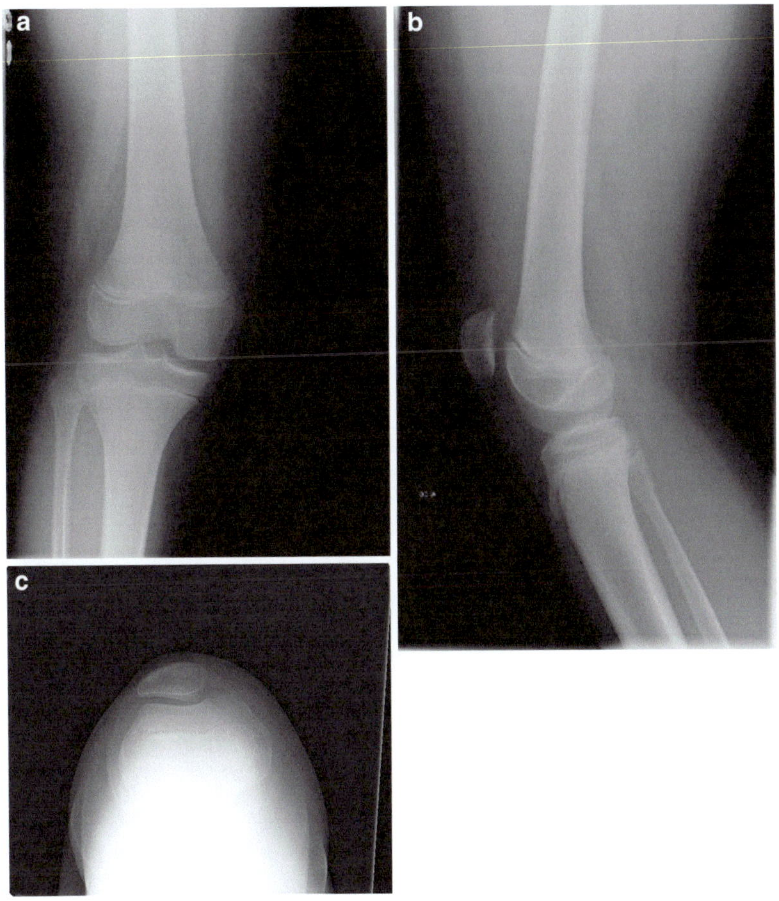

Fig. 4.2 Complete radiological examination of the patient of Fig. 4.1: anteroposterior view (**a**); lateral view (Insall-Salvati ratio of 1.7) (**b**); true skyline view of the patella (**c**)

Table 4.1 Recent literature for conservative versus surgical treatment of primary patellar dislocation

	Type of study	Number operative/ non-operative	Mean age	Follow-up mean years (range)	Redislocation rate (operative/ conservative) (%)	Observations
Nikku et al. [10]	Prospective randomised	70/57	20	7 (6–9)	31/39	Female, associated factors
Christiansen et al. [11]	Prospective randomised	80	20	2	17/20	Similar clinical outcome
Sillanpää et al. [12]	Prospective non-randomised	30/46	20	7	19/23	Operative better preinjury level
Sillanpää et al. [13]	Prospective randomised	18/22	20	7	0/28.5	Similar clinical outcome
Palmu et al. [14]	Prospective randomised	36/28	16	14	67/71	Good clinical outcome in both groups

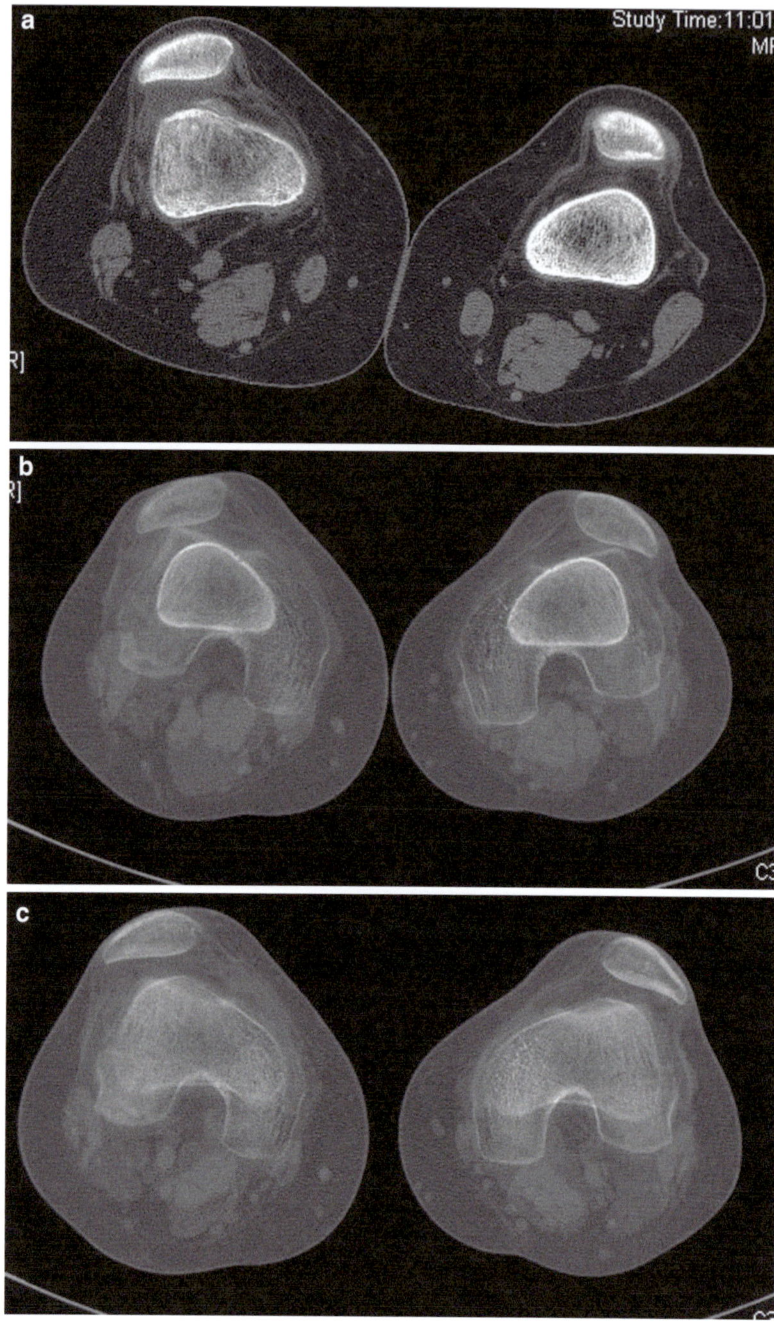

Fig. 4.3 Patellar CT (computed tomography) views of patient of Fig. 4.1. Injury of medial patellar soft tissue and medial patellofemoral ligament (**a**); measurement of version, torsion and trochlear angle (160°, normal 138°) (**b**); patellar subluxation with 20° of flexion of the knee (**c**)

preinjury level for the operative treatment in a non-randomised trial, however, the redislocation rate and overall results was again similar for both options [12]. The same group assessed and observed a lower redislocation rate for the surgical treatment in a randomised study, but they did not find any other clinical benefit for surgery [13]. Palmu et al. found a very high redislocation rate for both types of treatments in patients younger than 16-years old; however, the long-term clinical result was good for most patients [14].

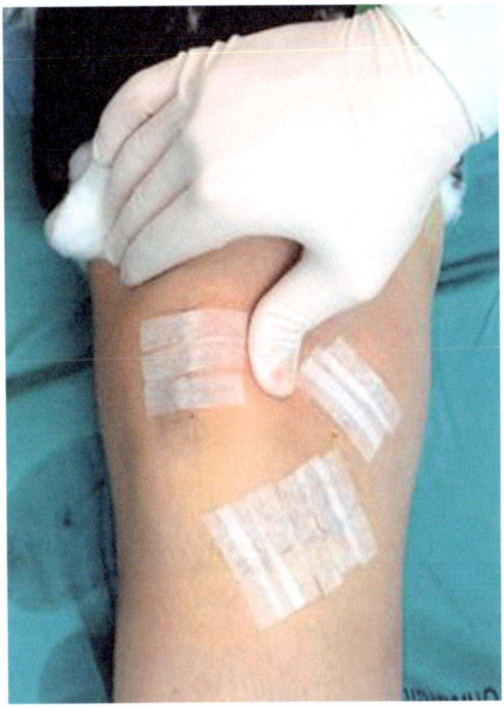

Fig. 4.4 Examination of the patella after surgical repair of medial patellofemoral ligament (MPFL)

Recent literature agrees that there is no a clear advantage for surgical treatment in primary patellar dislocation unless associated factors like previous episodes, contralateral lesions, trochlear dysplasia or high level of sport could determine this indication. To assess the anatomy of the knee in all patients after a primary dislocation of the knee a complete clinical (Q angle) and radiological study, including a computed tomography (CT) is required: patella height (Insall-Salvati technique), sulcus angle, patellar index, congruence angle, lateral patellofemoral angle and patellofemoral index [15] (Fig. 4.3). When operative treatment is the most appropriate option, reconstruction of the MPFL must be considered [16] (Fig. 4.4).

4.3 Osteochondral Fractures

Osteochondral fractures associated with dislocation of the patella are relatively frequent in adolescents: around one third of the patients with an acute dislocation may have bone lesions [17]. The mechanism of this injury is usually from a twist regarding the so-called flexion-rotation injury with compression and the associated patellar dislocation. The typical flexed knee after the traumatic event is observed at the Emergency Department and the aspiration reveals small fat globules in the blood. A fragment may be palpable as well as the feeling of a locking joint.

A careful evaluation of radiographs must be done in the three views (anteroposterior, lateral and axial) searching for every small fragment. Rorabeck and Bobechko observed three types of osteochondral fractures: an infero-medial patellar fracture; and the less common, lateral femoral condyle fracture, or the combination of both. If an ossified fragment is observed an MRI is indicated in order to assess the right size of the fragment.

Definite treatment depends on the size and the location of the fragment: a large fragment form a weight—bearing area need to be fixed, however, a small fragment from a non-weight bearing area may be excised. The latter are usually excised with arthroscopic surgery and have a good prognosis. Larger fragments, more than 1 cm, can be fixed by bicortical intraarticular screws or other hardware with good clinical and radiological results. For these lesions a careful examination of the knee is mandatory: for recurrent dislocation or subluxation predicts the prognosis of the injury, so, many surgeons advocate a repair of the medial structures, including the MPFL [18]. Regardless the method used for the fixation of the fragment all authors agree that enough, viable, non-sclerotic subchondral bone is needed to promote and adequate bone-to-bone healing [19]. It is also very important that patients need to be informed that complications like quadriceps insufficiency, adhesions or synovitis related to material can be observed.

4.4 Conclusions

Management for primary patellar dislocation must be conservative, however, a prior history of contralateral dislocation, anatomic disorders or patients with a high-level sport activity surgical treatment must be considered. Conservative treatment can be either immobilization in an above knee cast for 6 weeks or, more adequate with a careful evaluation, for 3 weeks in a splint, which allows immediate isometrics quadriceps activity. An adequate repair of the MPFL of the knee must be done when surgery is performed. When an osteochondral lesion is observed, a careful radiological evaluation (with CT and MRI) is recommended in order to assess the size and location of the bone fragment. The internal fixation of a large bone lesion provides a good result and a proper rehabilitation program.

References

1. Hawkins RJ, Bell RH, Anisette G (1986) Acute patellar dislocations: the natural history. Am J Sports Med 14:117–120
2. Stefancin JJ, Parker RD (2007) First-time traumatic patellar dislocations: a systematic review. Clin Orthop Relat Res 455:93–101
3. Wiberg G (1941) Roentgenographic and anatomic studies on the femoro-patellar joint. Acta Orthop Scand 12:319–410
4. Hautamaa PV, Fithian DC, Kaufman KR, Daniel DM, Pohlmeyer AM (1998) Medial soft tissue restraints in lateral patellar instability and repair. Clin Orthop Relat Res 349:174–182
5. Arnbjornsson A, Egund N, Rydling O, Stockerup R, Ryd L (1992) The natural history of recurrent dislocation of the patella: long-term results of conservative and operative treatment. J Bone Joint Surg Br 74:140–142
6. Waligora AC, Johanson NA, Hirsch BE (2009) Clinical anatomy of the quadriceps femoris and extensor apparatus of the knee. Clin Orthop Relat Res 467:3297–3306
7. Nomura E (1999) Classification of lesions of the medial patello-femoral ligament in patellar dislocation. Int Orthop 23:260–263
8. Maempaa H, Lehto MU (1997) Patellar dislocation. The long-term results of nonoperative management in 100 patients. Am J Sports Med 25:213–217
9. Monk AP, Doll HA, Gibbons CL, Ostlere S, Beard DJ, Gill HS, Murray DW (2011) The patho-anatomy of patellofemoral subluxation. J Bone Joint Surg Br 93:1341–1347
10. Nikku R, Nietosvaara Y, Aalto K, Kallio PE (2005) Operative treatment of primary patellar dislocation does not improve medium-term outcome. A 7-year follow-up report and risk analysis of 127 randomized patients. Acta Orthop 76:699–704
11. Christiansen SE, Jakobsen BW, Lund B, Lind M (2008) Isolated repair of the medial patellofemoral ligament in primary dislocation of the patella: a prospective randomized study. Arthroscopy 24:881–887
12. Sillanpää PJ, Mäenpää HM, Mattila VM, Visuri T, Pihlajamäki H (2008) Arthroscopy surgery for primary traumatic patellar dislocation: a prospective, nonrandomized study comparing patients treated with and without acute arthroscopic stabilization with a median 7-year follow-up. Am J Sports Med 36:2301–2309
13. Sillanpää PJ, Mattila VM, Mäenpää HM, Kiuru M, Visuri T, Pihlajamäki H (2009) Treatment with and without initial stabilizing surgery for primary traumatic patellar dislocation. A prospective, randomized study. J Bone Joint Surg Am 91:263–273
14. Palmu S, Kallio PE, Donell ST, Helenius I, Nietosvaara Y (2008) Acute patellar dislocation in children and adolescents: a randomized clinical trial. J Bone Joint Surg Am 90:463–470
15. Aglietti P, Insall J, Cerulli G (1983) Patellar pain and incongruence I. Measurements of incongruence. Clin Orthop Relat Res 176:217–221
16. Howells NR, Barnett AJ, Ahearn N, Ansari A, Eldrige JD (2012) Medial patellofemoral ligament reconstruction. J Bone Joint Surg Br 94:1202–1208
17. Nietosvaara Y, Aalto K, Kallio PE (1994) Acute patellar dislocation in children: incidence and associated osteochondral fractures. J Pediatr Orthop 14:513–515
18. Rorabeck CH, Bobechko WP (1976) Acute dislocation of the patella with osteochondral fracture. Review of 18 cases. J Bone Joint Surg Br 58:237–240
19. Bowers AL, Huffman GR (2008) Suture bridge fixation of a femoral condyle traumatic osteochondral defect. Clin Orthop Relat Res 466:2276–2281

5 Traumatic Knee Dislocation

E. Carlos Rodríguez-Merchán, Hortensia De la Corte-García, María Valencia-Mora and Primitivo Gómez-Cardero

5.1 Introduction

Traumatic knee dislocation (TKD) is an infrequent injury accounting for around 0.02 % of all the injuries to the musculoskeletal system [1–3] (Fig. 5.1). Misguided treatment of TKD is associated with serious consequences, especially in the presence of a vascular lesion (popliteal artery). This is the reason why, in spite of the low incidence of TKD, it is crucial to possess a clear understanding of the basic principles that should guide its treatment. TKD often damages most of the knee stabilizing tissues, which usually results in multi-directional knee joint instability. Although some dislocations affect only the anterior cruciate ligament (ACL) or the posterior cruciate ligament (PCL), in most cases both ligaments are torn. Associated injury to the medial or lateral collateral ligaments (MCL or LCL), the menisci, articular cartilage, or nerve structures (peroneal nerve) may further complicate treatment of TKD.

Many years ago, TKD used to be treated by long-term immobilization, but results were often unsatisfactory (loss of range of motion, residual instability, and poor joint function). At present, recommended treatment for TKR is surgical reconstruction (by means of allografts) of all ligament injuries combined with treatment of associated meniscal injuries (with partial meniscectomy or meniscal suture) [1–10]. Widespread use of allografts in multi-ligament knee surgery arises from the fact that they are easier to obtain, require less operating room time, and result in less morbidity to the donor site than autografts. Most authors recommend early reconstruction (at 3 weeks from injury) [11–22].

5.2 Classification

TKDs are classified into acute and chronic, depending on the length of time elapsed between injury and diagnosis (<3 and >3 weeks, respectively). The anatomical classification, on the other hand, is based on the direction of displacement of the tibia on the femur (anterior, posterior, medial, or lateral). A rotational knee dislocation involves displacement in two or more directions. TKDs that reduce spontaneously prior to diagnosis are classified according to the direction of instability [1–3].

The most frequent type of TKD is anterior dislocation (40 % of all TKDs); these are caused by hyperextension. Posterior dislocations account for 33 % of TKDs and are commonly produced

E. C. Rodríguez-Merchán (✉) · M. Valencia-Mora · P. Gómez-Cardero
Department of Orthopaedic Surgery, "La Paz" University Hospital-IdiPaz, Paseo de la Castellana 261, 28046, Madrid, Spain
e-mail: ecrmerchan@gmx.es

H. De la Corte-García
Department of Physical Medicine and Rehabilitation, "Doce de Octubre" University Hospital, Avenida de Córdoba s/n, 28041, Madrid, Spain

E. C. Rodríguez-Merchán (ed.), *Traumatic Injuries of the Knee*,
DOI: 10.1007/978-88-470-5298-7_5, © Springer-Verlag Italia 2013

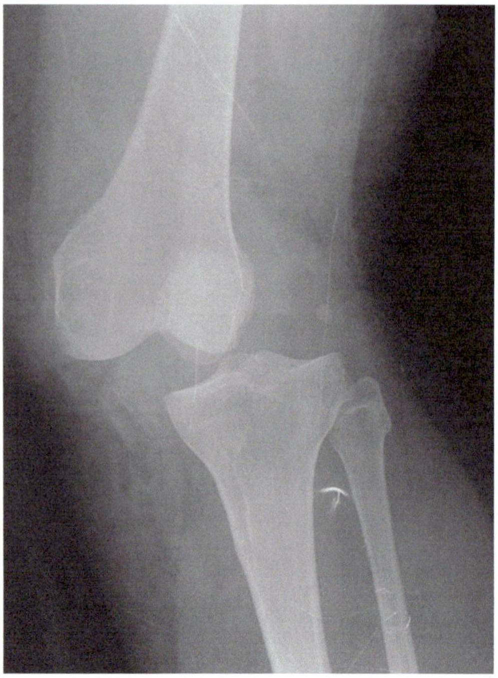

Fig. 5.1 Anteroposterior radiograph of a traumatic knee dislocation before it was reduced in the emergency department

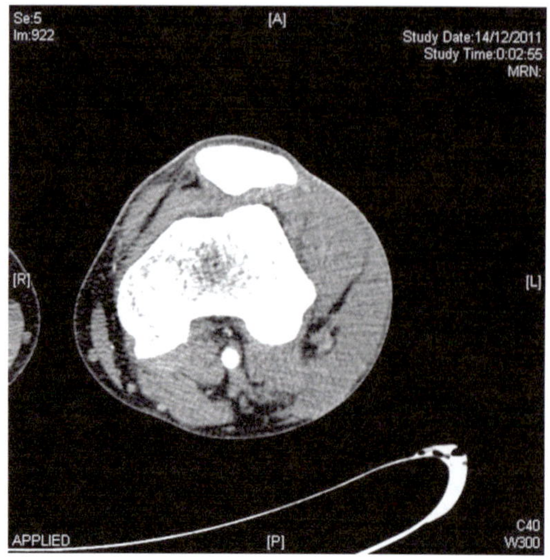

Fig. 5.2 An injury to the popliteal artery must always be ruled out in the presence of a traumatic knee dislocation. In this case, CT angiography revealed vasospasm and artery contusion, but as vascular flow was satisfactory severe vascular damage was ruled out. As a result, vascular surgery was deemed unnecessary

by high-energy trauma such as a dashboard injury in a car accident. Medial and lateral dislocations are less frequent, with an incidence of 4 and 18 %, respectively; the mechanism of injury is a large varus or valgus force. Rotational knee dislocations are the least common. The most frequently seen are posterolateral dislocations, which are extremely difficult to reduce as the medial femoral condyle perforates the soft tissues on the medial aspect of the joint [4–10].

5.3 Assessment

Initial assessment of TKD should begin with a detailed clinical history where the specific mechanism of injury must be investigated. Subsequently, a thorough physical examination should be performed, including a comprehensive neurovascular examination of the limb. Patients with TKD often complain of excruciating pain and present with large-scale joint effusion and diffuse inflammation in the limb involved. In multi-trauma patients, a spontaneously reduced TKD may go unnoticed. When there is significant laxity of two or more ligaments, the presence of TKD must be suspected [1–10].

Vascular examination must include palpation of arterial pulses (pedal and posterior tibial arteries), and comparison with the healthy side. The ankle-arm index, calculated by ultrasound, can help confirm the vascular status of the limb. A normal result does not rule out the existence of an arterial injury. Indeed, an arterial injury is compatible with a normal pulse rate, a warm foot, and seemingly adequate capillary filling. This means that patients with suspected TKD should be subjected to CT angiography (Fig. 5.2) or a lower limb arteriogram. Such tests are fully justified given their low morbidity, the high incidence of popliteal artery injury in these patients, and the serious consequences of diagnostic delay in these cases [9, 10].

It is also essential to conduct a comprehensive neurological assessment that includes the motor and sensory functions of the tibial and peroneal nerves. The risk of a compartment syndrome must not be underestimated [1–3].

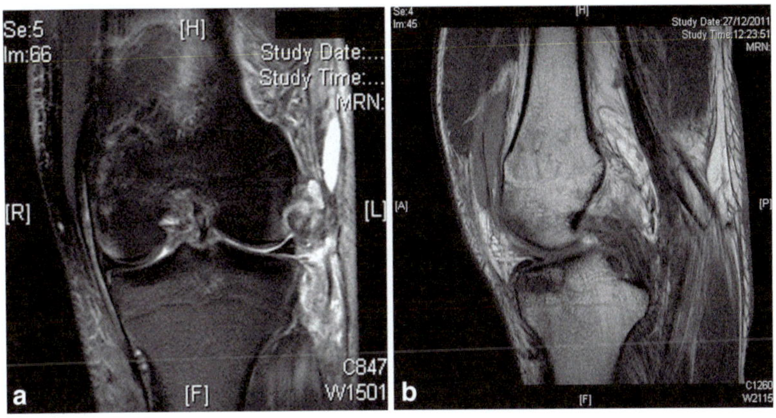

Fig. 5.3 (**a**) MRI of a patient with traumatic knee dislocation who also sustained a peroneal nerve injury. Anteroposterior view showing complete rupture of the LCL. (**b**) Lateral view exhibiting an ACL tear. In traumatic knee dislocation, one or both cruciate ligaments (ACL, PCL) may be injured together with one or both collateral ligaments (MCL, LCL). In this case, arthroscopic reconstruction of the ACL and open surgical reconstruction of the LCL were carried out using two Achilles tendon allografts. Both ligaments were reconstructed in a single surgical procedure at 3 weeks from injury

Evaluation of knee stability must only be carried out once the survival of the limb has been ensured. The assessment must be conducted with care so as not to cause potential iatrogenic injuries. It is often difficult to perform a thorough evaluation of the ligaments given the degree of pain often experienced by the patient. The Lachman test, carried out with the knee flexed at 30°, is the best method test to detect a deficient ACL. The most accurate way of identifying an injured PCL is the posterior drawer test, performed with the knee flexed at 90°. Integrity of the collateral ligaments (MCL, LCL) is assessed by applying forces on the coronal place, with the knee in full extension and at 30° of flexion.

Radiographs are necessary to determine the direction of dislocation, detect associated bone injuries (fracture or avulsion), and confirm reduction. Initial radiographs must be performed immediately after the clinical examination. An MRI (Magnetic Resonance Imaging) study must be carried out to identify associated bone or soft tissue injuries, but only once the patient has been stabilized. MRI is essential to chart the patient's surgical plan (Fig. 5.3).

5.4 Associated Vascular and Nerve Lesions

Injury to the popliteal artery could turn TKD into an emergency. The incidence of popliteal artery injury ranges between 32 and 45 % (from intimal tears to complete rupture of the artery). Taking into account that amputation rates vary in direct proportion with revascularization time, urgent detection of vascular compromise is of the essence. The rate of amputations is 86 % when revascularization is delayed between 6 and 8 h. Intimal injuries are at times particularly insidious, with manifestation of symptoms of vascular compromise occurring many days after their onset. In patients with TKD, a vascular lesion must be presumed as long as there is no CT angiographic or arteriographic evidence to the contrary.

Neurological lesions occur in 16–40 % of TKDs. Such lesions, which may range from the stretching of a nerve (neuropraxia) to its complete rupture (neurotmesis), are more common following posterolateral dislocation. The peroneal nerve is more often injured than the tibial nerve. Before manipulation of the knee, a comprehensive radiographic assessment is required. It must be noted, however, that performing such an assessment can be challenging, particularly in multi-trauma patients.

5.5 Initial Treatment

The vascular status of the involved limb must be urgently determined. If clear signs of ischemia are detected, the knee must immediately be reduced using gentle traction and counter-traction after administration of conscious sedation. Subsequently, the limb must be stabilized either with a long leg brace or, preferably, with an external fixator. Such a fixator is often rigid enough to keep the joint reduced and allows periodic inspections of both leg and knee. Should arterial pulses reappear following reduction, post-reduction radiographs and arteriography are required. If ischemia persists, an emergency surgical procedure will be needed to achieve revascularization. Following revascularization, a saphenous vein graft and a fasciotomy are often necessary to prevent a compartment syndrome. Emergency surgery is also indicated in the presence of compartment syndrome, open dislocation or irreducible dislocation. Regardless of whether TKD is present or not, diagnosis and early treatment of compartment syndrome are fundamental for a good result.

In open TKDs, it is essential to observe the basic principles of wound care (initial lavage and débridement followed by serial débridement if required), administer intravenous antibiotics, and provide appropriate soft tissue cover. Early ligament reconstruction (at 3 weeks) is contraindicated in open TKD. In some cases, problems related with soft tissue cover may delay ligament reconstruction for months.

Rare as they are, irreducible TKDs require immediate surgical reduction to avoid excessive traction of neurovascular structures. Although ligament reconstruction can be carried out at the same time as open reduction, it is best to defer the reconstruction until later so that a full imaging study (radiographs, MRI) and a comprehensive preoperative plan can be carried out.

5.6 Final Treatment

Treatment of multi-ligament knee injuries remains a significant challenge because of the multiple combinations of ligament and meniscus injuries that patients exhibit. Before 1975 non-surgical treatment was the norm, consisting of closed reduction followed by immobilization. The results of such treatment were not always satisfactory and greatly depended on the length of immobilization. If fact, longer immobilization resulted in stable, though stiff, knees whereas shorter immobilizations led to knees with excellent range of motion but substantial instability. Unfortunately, no prospective study has to date compared surgical with non-surgical treatment in these types of injuries. The latest advances in knee ligament surgery have made surgical treatment (ligament reconstruction at 3 weeks from injury) highly recommendable for patients with TKD. The purpose of surgery is to improve stability, preserve range of motion, and achieve a level of function that allows patients to perform their activities of daily living.

5.6.1 Nonsurgical Treatment

Although much used in the past, closed reduction and cast immobilization is only indicated at present in elderly or sedentary patients, or in those in extremely poor health. Patients initially treated non-surgically often require subsequent operations to resolve sequelae such as loss of range of motion and persistent instability. Poor results of conservative treatment of TKD are the norm.

Conservative treatment requires 6 weeks of knee immobilization in extension. Immobilization may be achieved by means of a plaster cast, a brace, external fixators, or transarticular Steinmann pins. In case of vascular repair, no casts or braces should be used to avoid circumferential pressures on the limb. An external fixator may

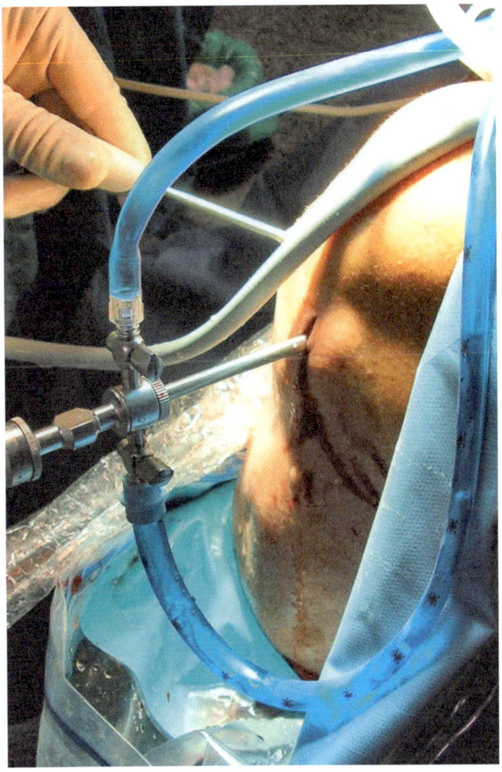

Fig. 5.4 Reconstruction of the cruciate ligaments was performed arthroscopically (same patient as in Fig. 5.3)

afford greater protection of vascularity. In grossly obese patients, it is often not possible to achieve immobilization just with a cast or a brace. Therefore, external fixators are also the most appropriate option for these patients.

The ideal flexion angle at which the dislocated knee should be immobilized is still a matter of debate. Taking into account that an ACL-deficient knee is more stable in flexion whereas a PCL-deficient knee is more stable in full extension, knee flexion between 30 and 45° would appear to be the most sensible alternative. Regardless of the immobilization angle chosen, the most important consideration is that the tibiofemoral joint should be appropriately reduced. With conservative treatment, frequent radiographs must be made, especially in the first few weeks, to make sure that the joint is still reduced. Immobilization, is followed by rehabilitation, which consists of progressive movements with the knee protected by a brace. This is followed by a gentle running program which, for most patients, can be introduced at 6–8 months.

5.6.2 Surgical Treatment

Most authors are against surgical treatment in patients with TKD. Normally, the best method to reestablish ligament stability as well as range of motion and overall function of the knee is simultaneous reconstruction of all existing injuries at 3 weeks from the initial lesion. The most common reconstructions are those of the ACL and/or the PCL, the collateral ligaments (MCL y/o LCL), and the capsule, particularly its posterolateral portion (Figs. 5.4, 5.5 and 5.6).

Performing the surgery after 3 weeks from injury has two main advantages. First, this period can be used to monitor vascular function and to resolve acute soft tissue inflammation. Second, range of motion and quadriceps tone will partially recover over these 3 weeks, which will decrease the risk of postoperative stiffness.

Nevertheless, a delay of more than 3 weeks may result in excessive scarring of the collateral ligaments and posterolateral structures, rendering them impossible to repair. If surgery needs to be delayed for over 3 weeks, it is best to wait for knee range of motion to improve. Late reconstruction should only be considered in cases of significant residual laxity and severe instability.

The type of lesion dictates the surgical approach to be used. The most common injuries are those affecting the ACL, PCL, and medial collateral ligament (MCL); and those affecting the ACL, PCL, lateral collateral ligament (LCL), and the posterolateral structures. A partially ruptured PCL does not need to be reconstructed. The type of injury will determine the location of skin incisions. Medial and lateral hockey-stick incisions, if separated at least 10 cm from each other, minimize the risk of skin necrosis and wound healing problems.

Several types of graft are available for ligament reconstruction. Depending on the extent of the injury, an autograft can be harvested from the ipsilateral or contralateral limb. Nevertheless, in

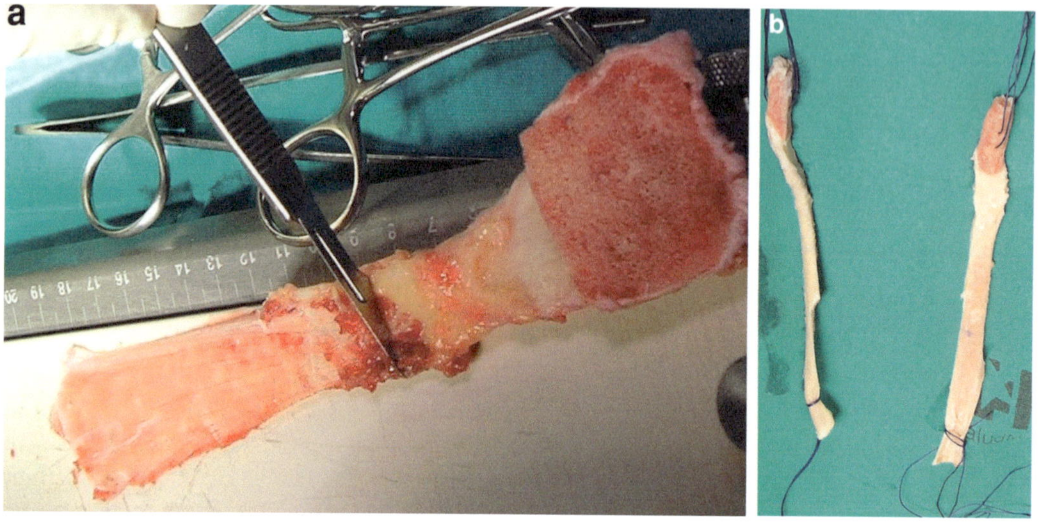

Fig. 5.5 View of the Achilles tendon allograft (**a**) before being divided into the two allografts (**b**) used to reconstruct the ACL and LCL (same patient as in Figs. 5.3 and 5.4)

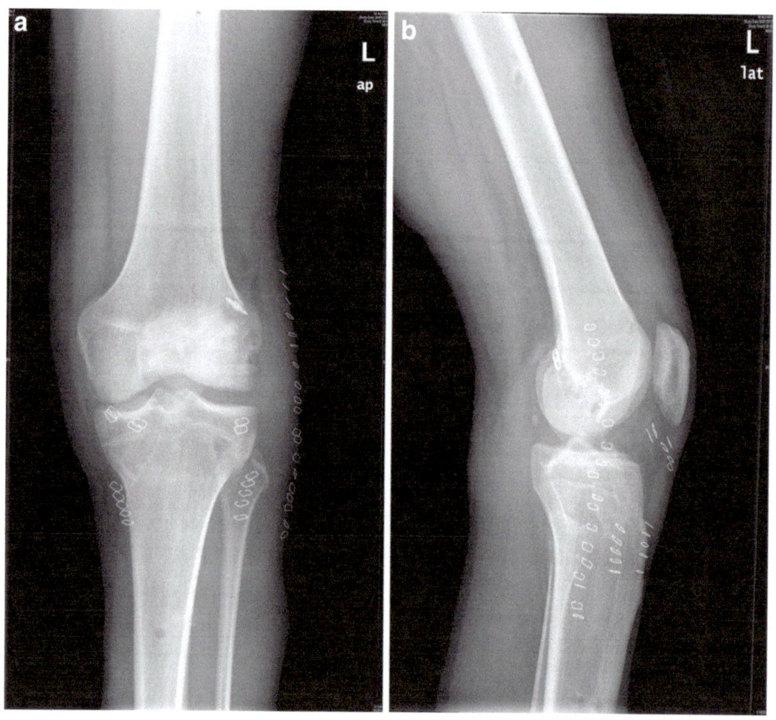

Fig. 5.6 Postoperative (**a**) anteroposterior and (**b**) lateral radiographs of the knee (same patient as in Figs. 5.3, 5.4 and 5.5) following arthroscopic ACL reconstruction and open surgical LCL reconstruction using two Achilles tendon allografts

knees with multiple ligament injuries allografts possess certain advantages over autografts. Use of allografts avoids the problem of donor site morbidity associated with autografts (Figs. 5.4, 5.5 and 5.6). Moreover, it reduces operating room time and the number and length of incisions needed in the injured knee. Use of allografts also reduces ischemia time and postoperative pain and stiffness. The disadvantages of allografts with respect to autografts include their higher price, the risk of disease transmission, and a slower incorporation and remodeling rates.

The technical details of cruciate ligament (ACL and PCL) reconstruction are well documented in the literature [1–22]. Arthroscopy is used to identify the tibial and femoral attachments of the cruciate ligaments. The PCL femoral tunnel must be placed so as to reproduce the anterolateral bundle of the native PCL, whereas the ACL tunnels should be placed at the center of the ligament's anatomical attachments.

In combined ACL-PCL-MCL injuries, where the lateral side opens up on full knee extension, a combined reconstruction must be made of the cruciates and the MCL (when examination under anesthesia with the knee in full extension reveals a grade III MCL injury). In patients with a grade III MCL injury, arthroscopic drilling of the cruciate ligament tunnels must be completed before proceeding to MCL repair.

A medial hockey-stick incision is made at the level of the vastus medialis, extending it over the femoral epicondyle to the anteromedial aspect of the tibia, just medially to the patellar tendon. In order to expose the MCL and the capsule, the sartorial fascia must be divided and reflected. Peripheral ruptures of the medial meniscus are repaired as part of the same approach by non-resorbable sutures. The MCL is repaired with non-resorbable sutures and bone anchors. MCL and capsule avulsions are repaired anatomically using bone anchors, whereas midsubstance MCL tears are repaired with non-resorbable 2/0 sutures using a modified Kessler stitch. In chronic situations, a reconstruction with semitendinosus or Achilles tendon allografts is required in addition to the suture repair. Both repair and reconstruction procedures are carried out with the knee flexed at 30°. To make sure that the knee will not lock, it must be continuously flexed and extended during the repair. The cruciate ligaments can then be fixed on the tibial side, as described above. Finally, a knee extension brace is applied.

In LCL injuries, a curved 12–18 mm incision is made over the lateral epicondyle. The starting point of this incision should be between the fibular head and the Gerdy tubercle. From here, the incision continues proximally over the lateral epicondyle until it reaches the posterior border of the posterior iliotibial tract. The peroneal nerve must now be identified and separated with a vessel loop. The simplest way to proceed is to locate the nerve proximally, behind the biceps femoris tendon, and follow it distally until it enters the anterior compartment of the leg. If a preoperative peroneal nerve injury is found, it must be documented. A formal neurolysis is not usually performed, although if a neurologic deficit is detected intraoperatively, the bundles of the fascia situated at the entrance to the anterior compartment will have to be released.

As regard the posterolateral structures, in acute cases both ligaments and tendons may be pulled off from their attachment. The surgeon must open the interval between the posterior border of the iliotibial tract and the biceps femoris tendon. Partial subperiosteal release of the attachment of the iliotibial tract from the Gerdy tubercle must also be performed in order to enlarge the exposure of the attachments of the LCL and the popliteal tendon. All repairs and reconstructions are made with the knee flexed at 30°.

Peripheral tears of the lateral meniscus are repaired with non-resorbable sutures, whereas capsular avulsions are fixed with bone anchors. LCL and popliteal tendon avulsions are anatomically repaired. An Achilles tendon allograft may be employed to reconstruct the LCL. Using an interference screw, a 7–8 mm bone block is fixed to the fibular head. The Achilles tendon allograft is fixed to the al lateral femoral epicondyle with bone anchors. The LCL stump must be carefully dissected so as to preserve its proximal and distal remnants. Such remnants must be tightened and then sutured to the Achilles tendon allograft, which will have previously been fixed to the lateral femoral condyle.

In the presence of an excessive preoperative posterolateral rotation, it is essential to address injuries to the popliteal tendon and to its several insertions. The location of the injury will determine the therapeutic method to be adopted. Femoral avulsions are sutured directly. In midsubstance injuries, a popliteal-peroneal reconstruction is performed with a hamstring tendon autograft, or a tibialis anterior tendon allograft. A tunnel is drilled in the proximal tibia. The graft is passed below the LCL and is placed in a blind tunnel in the area of the anatomical attachment of the popliteal tendon. The femoral insertion is now attached to a plastic button on the medial femoral cortex. The distal end is pulled out through the tunnel created in the fibular head and must then be tightened with the knee flexed at 30°. Fixation is achieved thanks to a resorbable interference screw positioned in the fibular head tunnel. In patients requiring a combined reconstruction of the LCL and the popliteal-peroneal ligament, the distal end of the popliteal-peroneal ligament is pulled forward through a soft tissue tunnel created at the attachment site of the biceps femoris tendon.

5.7 Residual Dislocation

Residual dislocation is a rare complication following surgery for TKD as patients are usually subjected to very strict follow-up protocols [23]. Two options are available to subjects who develop this complication: ligament reconstruction and total knee arthroplasty (TKA).

The authors have treated a woman who sustained a posterolateral TKD after being hit by a car. She was taken care of first by the intensive care unit, where she was diagnosed with pulmonary contusion, fracture of the nasal bones, and right-sided renal contusion. As she also exhibited an evident deformity in her left knee, she was referred to the orthopedic trauma department.

Physical examination demonstrated an evident valgus deformity in the left knee with posterior tibial displacement, suggesting a diagnosis of TKD. Distal vascular and nerve function were normal. The initial diagnosis of dislocation of the knee was confirmed by means of plain films. The dislocation was reduced under sedation and X-ray control, and the patient was immobilized with a long leg posterior splint to prevent the development of compartment syndrome. A follow-up X-ray exam carried out 5 days later revealed subluxation of the knee, which prompted the performance of an open reduction procedure with subsequent immobilization by external fixation. The surgical procedure revealed soft tissue entrapment in the lateral compartment, injury to both cruciate ligaments, detachment of the medial meniscus, which was reattached, and distension of both collateral ligaments. The results of successive follow-up exams being positive, the external fixator was removed at 2 weeks from surgery. The patient failed to keep her appointments for secondary ligament reconstruction.

Six years later, the patient presented again with functional inability to walk and disabling pain. Physical exploration revealed a deformed knee with frank anterior/posterior instability. The Lachman, pivot shift, and anterior and posterior drawer tests were all positive, as were varus and valgus stress tests at 0 and 30°. Lateral patellar dislocation was also identified. Radiographs confirmed the presence of chronic lateral subluxation of the knee, with concomitant lateral patellar dislocation and severe degenerative changes in all three compartments (Fig. 5.7). MRI demonstrated the absence of both cruciate ligaments, attenuation of the medial and lateral collateral ligaments, and serious degenerative changes compounded by a 14 mm bone defect in the medial portion of the tibia (Fig. 5.7).

In the face of this situation, implantation of a constrained TKR (CCK, Constrained Condylar Knee) in the left knee was decided. A medial parapatellar arthrotomy was performed with a straight midline incision. In order to facilitate range of motion and reduce the dislocation, an extensive release was carried out of both the medial and the lateral compartments as well as a resection of osteophytes and fibrous remnants from both cruciate ligaments. A tibial bone defect was identified that had been caused by impaction of the medial condyle. The posterior capsule was carefully detached from its insertion in the distal femur. On realizing that the CCK prosthesis was not providing enough stability, a rotating-hinge prosthesis (Waldemar Link^{R}) was implanted, with a 14 mm tibial extension stem. In order to correct the lateral patellar dislocation, it was necessary to recenter the patella by means of the Insall technique. Flexion of 100° was

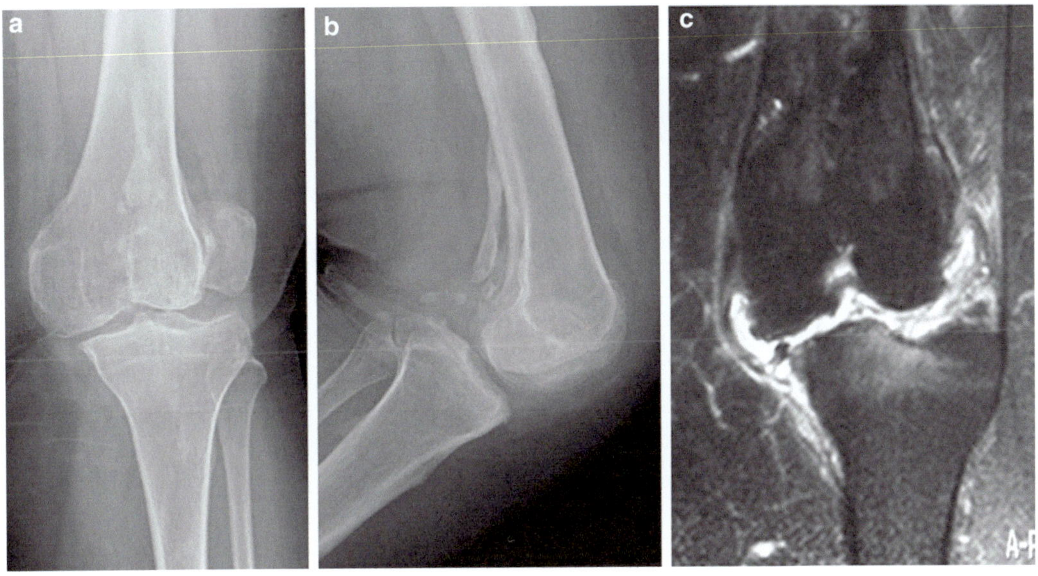

Fig. 5.7 49-year-old patient with a 6-year history of chronic subluxation who exhibited frank anterior/posterior and medial/lateral instability associated to severe degenerative changes. Anteroposterior X-ray (same image as in Fig. 5.1) of the right knee showed dislocation of the joint. Anteroposterior view of the knee taken 5 days after trauma showed subluxation of the knee inside the cast, confirming the instability of the injury. Six years after dislocation the anteroposterior (**a**) and lateral (**b**) views showed chronic subluxation of the knee with severe degenerative changes in the three joint compartments along with a lateral dislocation of the patella. Coronal view of a T2 MRI sequence (**c**) showed the attenuation of both lateral and medial collateral ligaments as well as the complete rupture of both cruciate ligaments. Severe destruction of the articular cartilage could also be seen

obtained intraoperatively with good patellar tracking through the entire range of motion. On the first day post-op, the patient was started on active range of motion exercises and on the seventh day from surgery, she exhibited an active and passive range of movement of 0–90°. Post-operative follow-up X-rays were satisfactory (Fig. 5.8).

Post-operative evolution was uneventful. At 2 years from surgery, the patient presented with full active and passive range of motion, without instability or pain. The prosthetic components still appeared to be well aligned and no signs of loosening were observed (Fig. 5.9).

Reduction with or without ligament repair or reconstruction has been used in recently sustained knee dislocations where the joint does not as yet exhibit any degenerative changes. Henshaw et al. reported on a case of chronic knee dislocation treated 24 weeks from injury by means of reduction and stabilization with Steinmann pins, without ligament repair or reconstruction [24]. At 22 months, the patient had a range of motion from 5 to 40° and was stable and pain-free. Nevertheless, other authors treating similar cases advocate the need to reconstruct the ligaments with allografts, maintaining the joint reduced by means of an external fixator until complete healing has occurred. Simonian et al. [25] reported on two cases of chronic posterior dislocation treated at 4 and 5 months from injury, where the ACL and PCL were repaired with an allograft and the posterolateral corner and the popliteal tendon were reconstructed with an Achilles tendon allograft. The patient was immobilized with an external fixator for 6 weeks with very good functional results in both instances at 1 year, with no recurrence of the previous instability.

Although ligament repair has provided favorable results in young patients with recently sustained chronic dislocations, joint replacement

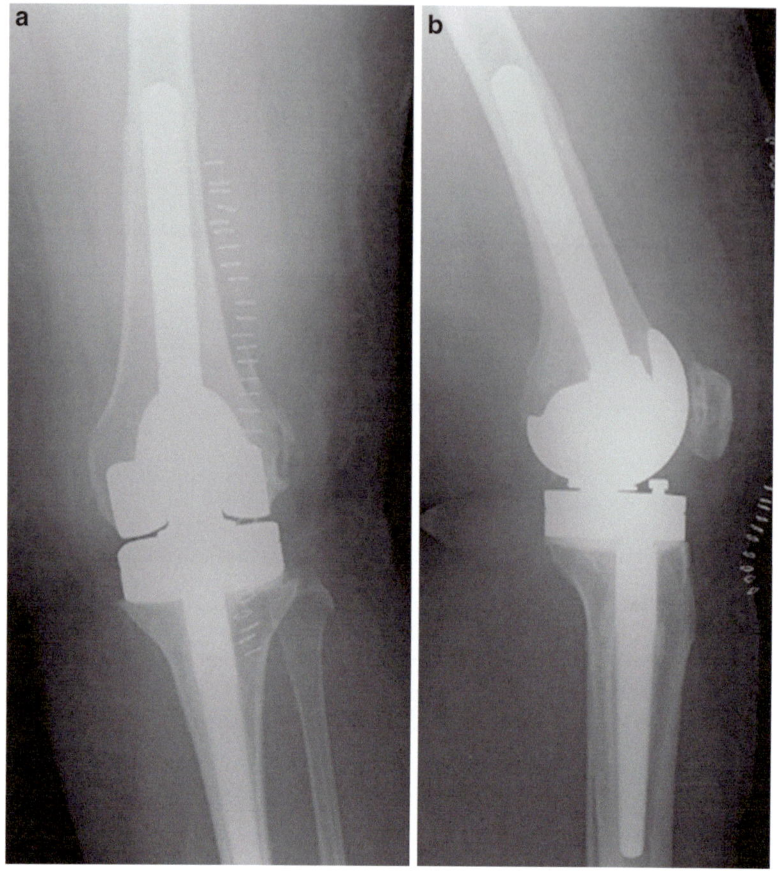

Fig. 5.8 Postoperative anteroposterior (**a**) and lateral (**b**) views of the same patient as in Fig. 5.7 showing the implanted rotating-hinge prosthesis

should be considered the treatment of choice in the presence of degenerative articular changes [26]. As we know, residual instability following TKD results in the development of degenerative changes in the joint, regardless of whether surgical or conservative treatment is administered. These changes are, however, more severe with non-surgical treatment [27, 28]. Conventional unconstrained TKAs have obtained poor functional results given the difficulties inherent in achieving prosthetic stability [29].

As mentioned above, most dislocations of the knee are accompanied by injury of at least three of the four major ligaments of the joint. In the face of a clinical situation characterized by tibiofemoral osteoarthritis compounded by ligament instability, it would seem advisable to employ prosthetic models that can afford greater stability: these can either be semiconstrained (CCK) or totally constrained (rotating-hinge prosthesis) [30, 31]. Petrie et al. [23] reported on two cases of chronic posterior subluxation successfully treated by an unconstrained TKR. The lateral collateral ligament was intact in both cases, which provided enough intraoperative stability. Liporace et al. [26] also reported on a case of a chronic posterolateral knee dislocation with 27 months' evolution that was treated with a semiconstrained prosthesis with long stems and superficial cementation of the tibial component. In this case, it was the medial collateral ligament that was intact.

5.8 Evidence-Based Medicine

One-third of TKDs that present at the Emergency Department are unreduced [32]. Approximately 25 % of TKD cases exhibit normal bone alignment on radiographic examination. In

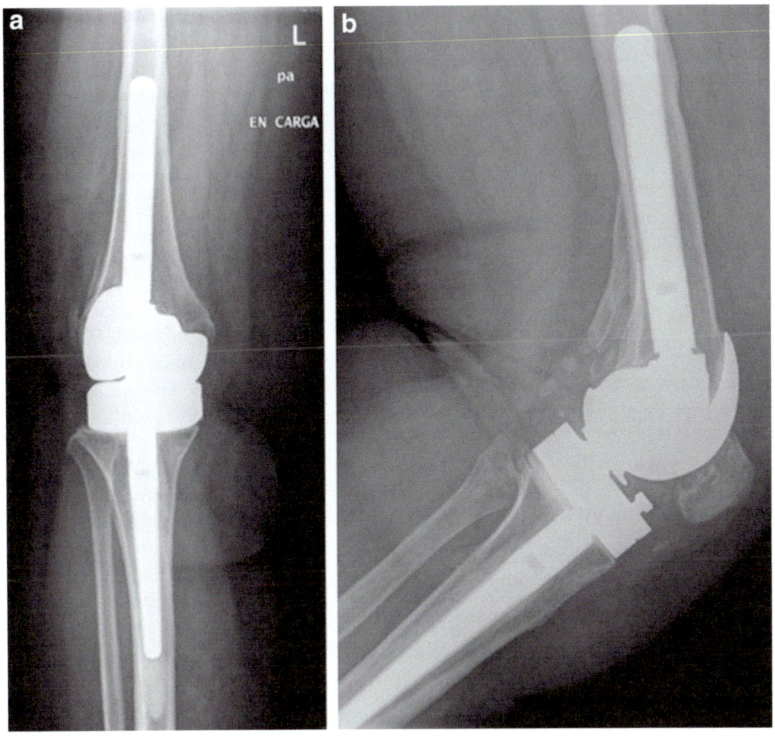

Fig. 5.9 Anteroposterior (**a**) and lateral (**b**) views of the same patient as in Figs. 5.7 and 5.8 showing the rotating-hinge prosthesis 2 years after surgery

addition, one-third of TKDs are not even suspected when an MRI is requested. It should be remembered that one, two, three, or all four ligaments of the knee (MCL, LCL, ACL, and PCL) may be ruptured. It is essential that TKD should be detected as soon as possible.

As regard the management of TKD, it has been shown that surgical treatment provides better functional results, greater stability, and is associated with a lower risk of developing joint stiffness than non-surgical treatment. It is important to reconstruct the posteromedial and posterolateral corners (with allografts). Early or acute (at 3 weeks from injury) suturing of the damaged ligaments has been associated with a lower failure rate (0–16 %) than late (chronic) repair, whose failure rate stands between 29 and 66 %. With respect to reconstruction, the so-called acute reconstruction (at 3 weeks) provides better results than chronic reconstruction. Reconstruction of the injured ligaments is associated with a failure rate of 2 %, whereas repair of those ligaments fails in 17 % of cases [32].

As far as prognosis is concerned, the incidence of knee stiffness following dislocation is of up to 19 %, although this figure has recently gone down as a result of the use of modern reconstruction and postoperative rehabilitation techniques. Even in successful reconstructions, between 17 and 22 % of patients go on to develop instability, which is an indication that the problem has not been fully resolved. Although patients with TKD can usually go back to their previous job, they seldom manage to regain their prior sport activity level [32].

5.9 Conclusions

TKD is a relatively infrequent injury. Nonetheless, taking into account its seriousness and the severe complications it could cause, it is essential to diagnose and treat it as early as possible. Diagnosis should include an adequate clinical history, a comprehensive examination of both the ligaments, and the neurovascular structures as well as certain imaging studies such as radiographs and MRI. If there is a suspicion of TKD, a CT angiography and/or an arteriogram must be carried out to rule out a potential injury to the popliteal artery. Initial treatment must be provided immediately by means of closed reduction and external fixation. After treatment, it is required to once again assess the neurovascular status of the limb and perform new radiographs to confirm that reduction has been successful. In patients with an open dislocation, compartment syndrome, a vascular lesion, or irreducible dislocation, emergency open surgery is indicated.

Treatment of a TKD with multiple ligament injuries should include ACL and PCL allograft reconstruction at 3 weeks from initial injury. During the same procedure, the surgeon must use allografts to reconstruct full-thickness injuries of the LCL and any damaged posterolateral structures. Although this type of surgery is highly demanding from a technical standpoint, ligament reconstruction can provide adequate knee stability, an acceptable range of motion and satisfactory joint function. Postoperative rehabilitation is also essential for success.

Patients with TKD usually have associated meniscal and osteochondral injuries, which tend to complicate treatment. When TKD is suspected, an arteriogram and/or a CT angiography must be performed to assess the vascular status of the limb.

References

1. Montgomery JB (1987) Dislocation of the knee. Orthop Clin North Am 18:149–156
2. Good L, Johnson RJ (1995) The dislocated knee. J Am Acad Orthop Surg 3:284–292
3. Brautigan B, Johnson DL (2000) The epidemiology of knee dislocations. Clin Sports Med 19:387–397
4. Walker DN, Rogers W, Schenck RC Jr (1994) Immediate vascular and ligamentous repair in a closed knee dislocation: case report. J Trauma 36:898–900
5. Tsiagadigui JG, Sabri F, Sintzoff S, Schuind F (1997) Magnetic resonance imaging for irreducible posterolateral knee dislocation. J Orthop Trauma 11:457–460
6. Cole BJ, Harner CD (1999) The multiple ligament injured knee. Clin Sports Med 18:241–262
7. Stayner LR, Coen MJ (2000) Historic perspectives of treatment algorithms in knee dislocation. Clin Sports Med 19:399–413
8. Wascher DC (2000) High-velocity knee dislocation with vascular injury treatment principles. Clin Sports Med 19:457–477
9. Rihn JA, Groff YJ, Harner CD, Cha PS (2004) The acutely dislocated knee: evaluation and management. J Am Acad Orthop Surg 12:334–346
10. Klineberg EO, Crites BM, Flinn WR, Archibald JD, Moorman CT 3rd (2004) The role of arteriography in assessing popliteal artery injury in knee dislocations. J Trauma 56:786–790
11. Giannoulias CS, Freedman KB (2004) Knee dislocations: management of the multiligament-injured knee. Am J Orthop 33:553–559
12. Kurtz CA, Sekiya JK (2005) Treatment of acute and chronic anterior cruciate ligament-posterior cruciate ligament-lateral side knee injuries. J Knee Surg 18:228–239
13. Cummings JR, Pedowitz RA (2005) Knee instability: the orthopaedic approach. Semin Musculoskelet Radiol 9:5–16
14. Helgeson MD, Lehman RA Jr, Murphy KP (2005) Initial evaluation of the acute and chronic multiple ligament injured knee. J Knee Surg 18:213–219
15. Tzurbakis M, Diamantopoulos A, Xenakis T, Georgoulis A (2006) Surgical treatment of multiple knee ligament injuries in 44 patients: 2–8 years follow-up results. Knee Surg Sports Traumatol Arthrosc 14:739–749
16. Robertson A, Nutton RW, Keating JF (2006) Dislocation of the knee. J Bone Joint Surg Br 88:706–711
17. Shelbourne KD, Haro MS, Gray T (2007) Knee dislocation with lateral side injury: results of an en masse surgical repair technique of the lateral side. Am J Sports Med 35:1105–1117
18. Patterson BM, Agel J, Swiontkowski MF, Mackenzie EJ, Bosse MJ LEAP Study Group (2007) Knee dislocations with vascular injury: outcomes in the Lower Extremity Assessment Project (LEAP) study. J Trauma 63:855–858
19. Stefancin JJ, Parker RD (2007) First-time traumatic patellar dislocation: a systematic review. Clin Orthop Relat Res 455:93–101
20. Bin SI, Nam TS (2007) Surgical outcome of 2-stage management of multiple knee ligament injuries after knee dislocation. Arthroscopy 23:1066–1072
21. Ricchetti ET, Sennett BJ, Huffman GR (2008) Acute and chronic management of posterolateral corner injuries of the knee. Orthopedics 31:479–488
22. Seroyer ST, Musahl V, Harner CD (2008) Management of the acute knee dislocation: the Pittsburgh experience. Injury 39:710–718
23. Petrie RS, Trousdale RT, Cabanela ME (2000) Total knee arthroplasty for chronic posterior knee

dislocation: report of two cases with technical considerations. J Arthoplasty 15:380–386
24. Henshaw RM, Saphiro MS, Oppenheim WL (1996) Delayed reduction of traumatic knee dislocation. A case report and literature review. Clin Orthop Relat Res 330:152–156
25. Simonian PT, Wickiewicz TL, Hotchkiss RN, Warren SF (1998) Chronic knee dislocation: reduction, reconstruction and application of a skeletally fixed knee hinge. A report of two cases. Am J Sports Med 26:591–596
26. Liporace FA, Hommen JP, Su ET, Jeong GK, Dayan AJ (2006) Semiconstrained knee arthroplasty in the setting of a chronic knee dislocation. A case report. J Orthop Trauma 20:286–288
27. Taylor AR, Arden GP, Rainey HA (1972) Traumatic dislocation of the knee: A report of forty-three cases with special reference to conservative treatment. J Bone Joint Surg Br 54:96–102
28. Karataglis D, Bisbinas I, Green MA, Learmonth DJ (2006) Functional outcome following reconstruction in chronic multiple ligament deficient knees. Knee Surg Sports Traumatol Arthrosc 14:843–847
29. Chen H-C, Chiu F-Y (2007) Chronic knee dislocation treated with arthroplasty. Injury Extra 38:258–261
30. Parsley BS, Sugano N, Bertolusso R, Conditt MA (2003) Mechanical alignment of tibial stems in revision total knee arthroplasty. J Arthroplasty 18:33–36
31. McAuley JP, Engh GA (2003) Constraint in total knee arthoplasty: when and what? J Arthroplasty 18:592–599
32. Stannard JP, Hammond A (2012) Knee dislocations. In: Bhandari M (ed) Evidence-based Orthopedics. Wiley-Blackwell, Oxford, pp 527–553

Floating Knee

6

Fernando Oñorbe-San Francisco and E. Carlos Rodríguez-Merchán

6.1 Introduction

Floating knee is the result of simultaneous ipsilateral fracture of the femur and tibia, disconnecting the knee from the rest of the extremity. This type of injury was first described by Blake and McBryde in 1975 [1], and comprises both diaphyseal fractures of the femur and tibia, and articular fractures. In children, fractures through the growth plate of the distal femur or of the proximal tibia can also give rise to floating knee.

Injuries of this kind are infrequent, though the increase in prevalence of high-energy trauma has caused a rise in the number of cases of floating knee. As is usually seen in severe trauma, the incidence of floating knee is greater in young male patients. The largest series published to date is that of Kao et al. [2], who analyzed 419 cases, of which 70.4 % corresponded to males. The most frequent range of age was 10–30 years.

Floating knee is a high-energy injury most often caused by traffic accidents (automobile, motorcycle or pedestrians or cyclists who are run over) [3]. Floating knee can also be caused by falls from a height or working accidents. The combination of ipsilateral fracture of the femur and tibia is a severe injury that usually also affects vital organs, with abundant musculoskeletal damage.

The present chapter reviews the most important aspects of floating knee: its classification, the associated lesions, its evaluation and prognostic factors, management, treatment outcome, and complications.

6.2 Classification

The classification of floating knee can be complicated, as reflected by the abundance of classifications proposed for such a not very frequent type of injury. The fact that classification is required of the fractures of two different bones, each of which may possess very distinct characteristics (one open and the other closed, one of an articular nature and the other diaphyseal) is what makes classification consensus difficult.

Blake and McBryde proposed a classification system based on joint involvement of the fractures [1]. In this context, type I fractures or "true floating knee" correspond to those cases in which neither fracture presents joint involvement at knee level. In turn, type II fractures or "false floating knee" correspond to those cases

F. Oñorbe-San Francisco (✉)
Department of Orthopaedic Surgery, Hospital Universitario Infanta Leonor, Gran Vía del Este 80, 28031, Madrid, (Madrid), Spain
e-mail: dronorbe@gmail.com

E. C. Rodríguez-Merchán
Department of Orthopaedic Surgery, "La Paz" University Hospital-IdiPaz, Paseo de la Castellana 261, 28046, Madrid, Madrid, Spain
e-mail: ecrmerchan@gmx.es

E. C. Rodríguez-Merchán (ed.), *Traumatic Injuries of the Knee*,
DOI: 10.1007/978-88-470-5298-7_6, © Springer-Verlag Italia 2013

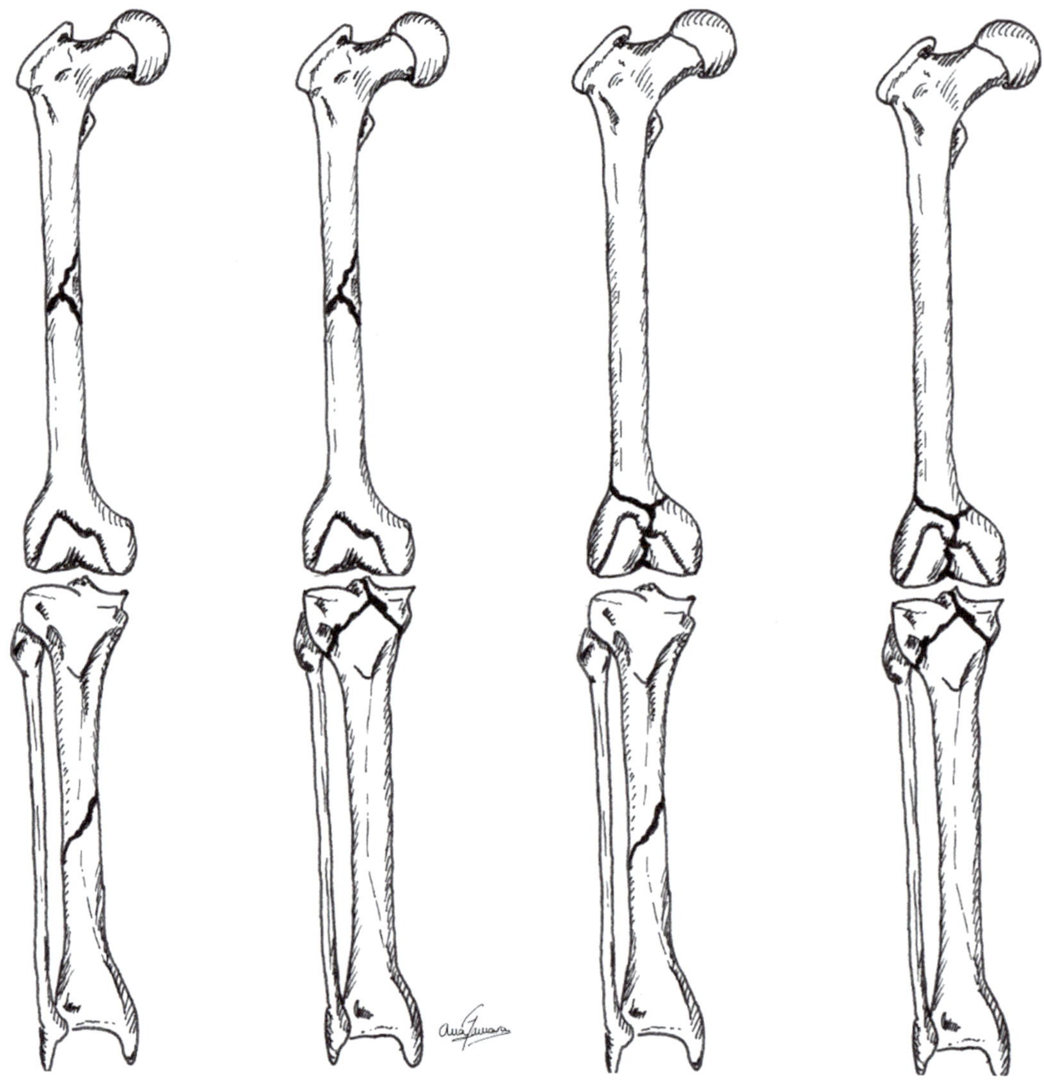

Fig. 6.1 Floating knee classification of Fraser et al. [4]

in which one of the two fractures affects the joint surface.

Three years later, Fraser et al. [4] (Fig. 6.1) modified the classification of Blake and McBryde by including three subtypes within type II. Type IIA corresponds to femoral diaphyseal fracture associated to fracture of the tibial plateau; type IIB involves distal femoral joint fracture with tibial diaphyseal fracture; and type IIC corresponds to articular fracture of both bones.

Letts et al. introduced a new classification (Fig. 6.2) applicable to pediatric fractures, though some authors have used it in adult patients, where its validity may be similar [5]. The novelty of this classification is that it assesses fractures not only as joint or diaphyseal injuries but also as open or closed fractures. Five types of fractures are described: type A fractures are closed diaphyseal fractures of both bones; type B cases comprise diaphyseal fracture of one bone and metaphyseal fracture of the other, both

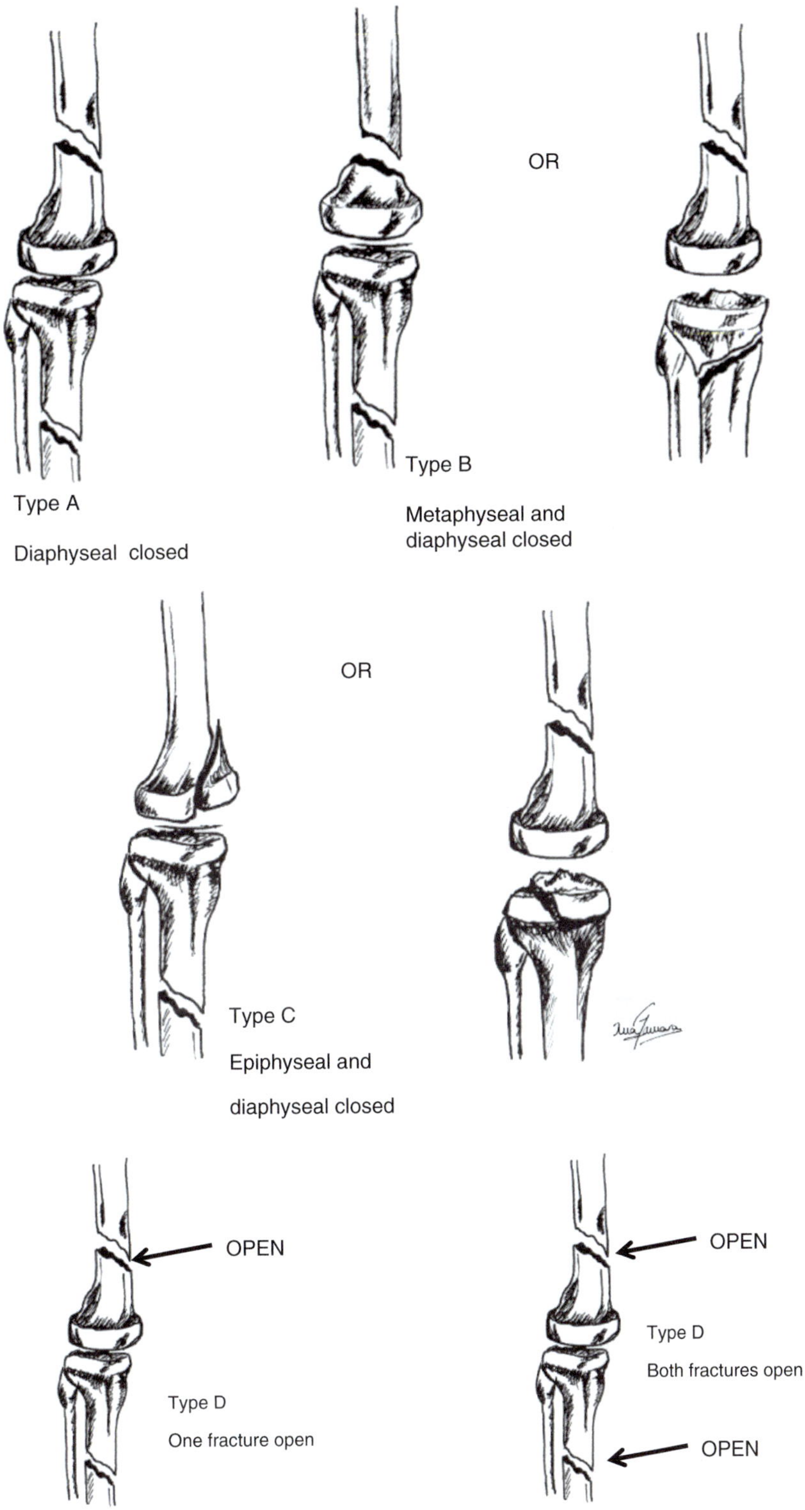

Fig. 6.2 Floating knee classification of Letts et al. [5]

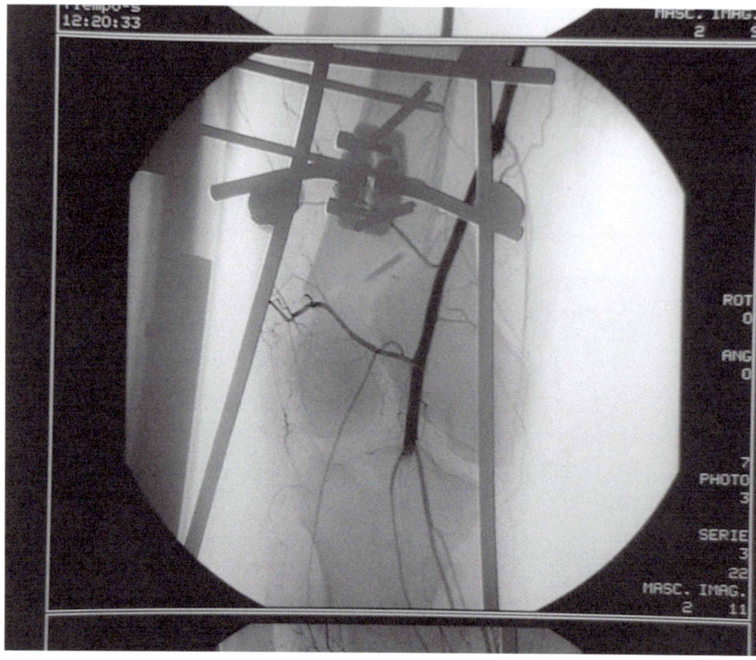

Fig. 6.3 Complete popliteal arterial damage in a case of floating knee

closed; type C fractures correspond to diaphyseal fracture of one bone and epiphyseal fracture of the other, both closed also; type D fracture is characterized by open fracture of one of the two bones; and type E fractures involve open fractures of both bones, regardless of their location.

In 1991, Bohn and Durbin, in a review of pediatric patients, used a classification similar to that of Fraser et al. in adults, but obviating the presence of open or closed fractures. As a result, only three types of fractures were considered [6]: type I (diaphyseal fractures), type II (at least one juxta-articular fracture), and type III (at least one epiphysiolysis).

Lastly, Arslan et al. modified the classification of Bohn, leaving fracture types I and II without changes [7]. Type III fractures were subdivided into type IIIa (involving a single physeal lesion) and type IIIb (with epiphysiolysis of both bones). These authors in turn introduced type IV fractures, including bifocal fractures of at least one of the two bones.

6.3 Associated Injuries

Patients with ipsilateral fracture of the femur and tibia are polytraumatized individuals that usually present more serious associated lesions than patients with isolated femoral or tibial fractures. In fact, the diagnosis of floating knee intrinsically implies a diagnosis of polytraumatism, since the latter is defined as the presence of two or more serious traumatisms (in this case of the tibia and femur). The incidence of associated life-threatening injuries reportedly reaches 74 % [4] [8], and the severity of these associated injuries is reflected by the mortality rate (5–15 %). Important bleeding is frequent, causing hypovolemic shock in a significant number of cases, as well as fat embolism in the first hours after trauma. In a series of 54 patients published by Veith et al., 7 cases of fat embolism (13 %), three pulmonary embolisms, and one death were recorded [9].

The series published by Kao et al. documents the associated lesions and complications in 419 patients with floating knee [2]. Of these subjects, 261 (62.3 %) have associated injuries, the most frequent locations being other extremities (54.9 %), head injuries (26.3 %), and pelvic damage (8.8 %).

Vascular damage in the vicinity of floating knee has been reported in 5–29 % of the cases [8], affecting particularly the posterior tibial artery. Vascular damage in turn is most often associated with intraarticular fractures [10] (Fig. 6.3). Arterial damage is the main reason for the high frequency of amputation of the affected extremity in these patients. It can also give rise to compartment syndrome, which nevertheless is a relatively rare complication in patients of this kind. The incidence was found to be 1.4 % in the series published by Fraser et al. [4].

The peroneal nerve is the most commonly affected peripheral nerve, with less frequent involvement of the sciatic nerve [3]. Such cases often correspond to neurapraxia, followed by spontaneous complete recovery, though genuinely irreversible nerve lesions with permanent sequelae are not infrequent.

Damage to the ligaments of the affected knee is very common. Szalay et al. reported a 53 % incidence of clinical laxity, versus an incidence of only 27 % in the case of patients with isolated femoral fracture [11]. However, lesions with an impact upon knee stability were much less common (close to 18 %)—the most frequent presentation being anterolateral instability. Meniscal rupture has been recorded in a large percentage of cases in which magnetic resonance imaging (MRI) has been performed on a systematic basis. However, such meniscal damage is usually asymptomatic. Concomitant damage to the anterior cruciate ligament (ACL) has been reported in 5–39 % of the cases [12, [13].

The high energy involved in such fractures produces extensive soft tissue damage, with a high incidence of open fractures (much higher than in series of isolated femoral or tibial fractures). In effect, between 58 and 81 % of these injuries are open fractures, with a predominance of tibial fractures [8, 9].

6.4 Evaluation

Patients with ipsilateral fracture of the femur and tibia have generally suffered polytraumatism and thus require advanced life-support measures. In addition, damage to other vital organs must be identified and treated, and admission to Intensive Care may prove necessary. The general condition of the patient may require the activation of Damage Control protocols, with provisional fracture stabilization using external fixation, or early definitive treatment [14].

Regarding osteoarticular exploration, a thorough evaluation is required of the ipsilateral hip, foot, and ankle in order to discard associated injuries which are not infrequent. Veith et al. described 12 ipsilateral foot and ankle and three ipsilateral hip injuries in a series of 53 floating knees [9].

Early and careful neurovascular exploration is needed, with the use of all necessary complementary tests in the case of diagnostic doubt. The advisability of systematic arteriographic study of patients with injuries of this kind is controversial. The presence of open fractures or compartment syndrome must be ruled out from the start.

The X-ray study should be made in two projections, including the joint proximal and distal to the fracture. Some joint fractures, such as tibial pilon or plateau fracture, may require computed tomography (CT) in order to establish a correct diagnosis.

6.5 Prognostic Factors

In 2001, Hee et al. reviewed their experience in 89 patients diagnosed with floating knee, conducting a multivariate statistical analysis of the factors associated with a poor prognosis and the appearance of complications [15]. The factors related to a poor outcome were older age, smoking, a high initial ISS (index severity score), open fractures, and comminuted fractures.

Based on these data, the authors developed a preoperative prognostic scale predicting the outcome with a sensitivity of 72 % and a specificity of 90 %.

Likewise, Hung et al. [16] reported poorer results in patients presenting intraarticular fractures with involvement of the knee joint (type IIA of Blake and McBryde classification [1] compared with patients with extraarticular fractures (type I) or intraarticular fractures with involvement of the hip or ankle (type IIB).

6.6 Treatment

Relatively few studies on this type of injury have been published to date. As a result, there are no universally accepted treatment principles. Moreover, the existing studies generally involve few cases, with a heterogeneous group of lesions documented over long periods of time.

Controversy remains regarding the optimum method and timing of treatment. Management of the fractures includes techniques as diverse as closed reduction and plaster, skeletal traction, and internal or external fixation, in both the femur and the tibia. The chosen method depends on the systemic patient conditions, the soft tissue conditions, the type of fracture, the availability of implants, and the experience and preferences of the surgeon.

6.6.1 Timing of Treatment

Patients with ipsilateral fractures of the femur and tibia often require advanced life-support measures. Consequently, the timing of fracture stabilization must be integrated in the context of multidisciplinary management of the polytraumatized individual. Open fractures, those with vascular damage, and fractures with a high risk of compartment syndrome or with established compartment syndrome, constitute orthopedic emergencies. In any case, the polytraumatized patient must undergo fracture stabilization as soon as possible in order to improve the prognosis.

The stabilization of intraarticular fractures can be postponed a few days until the soft tissue swelling has decreased, since tibial plateau and pilon fractures often involve significant skin and soft tissue damage, and in this context delayed treatment may result in fewer complications and an improved outcome.

6.6.2 Conservative Treatment

The non-surgical management of ipsilateral fractures of the femur and tibia was common practice in the 1960s and 1970s, but the results were not satisfactory. Blake and McBryde used non-surgical treatment in 26 of the 37 femoral fractures and in all 37 of the tibial fractures in their series [1]. Most of the patients had some permanent functional disability, chronic pain and limping. As a result of this study, surgery of at least one of the two fractures began to be advised.

Starting in the late 1970s, intramedullary femoral fixation became the most widely accepted treatment option. Floating knee was no exception to this practice, and began to be treated with femoral nailing and plastering of the tibial fracture. At present, it is clear that the best treatment option for these injuries is surgery of both fractures, except in some isolated cases of non-displaced tibial fracture. In 1984, only 9 years after the study published by Blake and McBryde, Veith et al. presented a series of 57 cases in which 56 femoral fractures and close to one-half of the tibial fractures were subjected to surgery [9]. Good or excellent results were obtained in 80 % of the cases, with a mean knee mobility range of 129 degrees.

6.6.3 Surgical Treatment

As we have mentioned, the currently recommended treatment for floating knee is surgical fixation of both fractures. It has been shown in both adults [9, 17] and in children [18] that although these initially are more serious cases, surgery of both fractures results in a better outcome, with fewer complications and reoperations (without counting removal of the osteosynthesis material), a shorter hospital stay, and a faster return to normal activity.

There are several surgical options for each of the fractures, and the indication should be conditioned by a series of factors such as the fracture pattern, the degree of soft tissue involvement, the associated lesions, and the surgeon's preference.

The use of external fixation is essential for the initial management of these patients, and in some cases it may be maintained as definitive treatment. Rooser and Hansson published a series of five patients subjected to external fixation of both fractures as definitive treatment, with no incidence of nonunion [19]. However, infection of the pin trajectory was recorded in three cases, with knee stiffness in three patients. It is well known that external fixation in femoral fractures can cause such mobility defects secondary to fixation of the quadriceps muscle. The authors themselves do not recommend the routine use of external fixation of the femur, and advise intramedullary nailing in such cases.

Likewise, Behr et al. published a series of six cases subjected to flexible intramedullary Ender nailing of both fractures; only one patient presented nonunion (of both bones), and the results were excellent or good in four patients [20]. The series was very small, however, and firm conclusions therefore cannot be drawn.

Surgical advances have influenced the treatment of these fractures. The use of retrograde femoral and antegrade tibial nails allows simultaneous surgical management of both fractures through a single incision. Many authors have reported good results with retrograde femoral nailing. Gregory et al. reviewed a series of 26 floating knees subjected to retrograde femoral nailing and anterograde tibial nailing without reaming, through a single incision [21]. Excellent results were obtained in 13 cases and acceptable results in 7, with a mean knee range of movement of 120°. Ostrum in turn reviewed 17 cases treated through a single 4-cm incision [22]. Five cases of nonunion were recorded in the 34 fractures of his series. Only one patient suffered knee stiffness, and none experienced postoperative pain. Good or very good final results were obtained in 88 % of patients (15 of the 17 cases). The use of a single incision can shorten surgery time and the trauma associated to surgery, mainly in cases with significant skin and soft tissue damage.

An inconvenience of retrograde intramedullary femoral nailing is that it complicates subsequent treatment of the frequent cruciate ligament damage, observed in up to 53 % of cases, according to Szalay et al. [11]. Thus, some authors recommend anterograde nailing of both fractures [23] (Fig. 6.4).

6.6.4 Treatment of Pediatric Floating Knee

The literature on pediatric floating knee is much more limited, since such injuries are even less common in the pediatric population. The first authors to publish a series exclusively involving patients under 15 years of age were Letts et al., in 1986, who introduced a new classification with implications for treatment [5]. In type A fractures (diaphyseal fractures of both bones), these authors recommend open reduction and fixation of the tibial fracture and skeletal traction of the femur. In type B injuries (one metaphyseal fracture), they use open reduction and fixation of the diaphyseal fracture and traction or plaster applied to the metaphyseal fracture. On the other hand, in type C fractures (one epiphysiolysis and one diaphyseal fracture), they recommend open reduction and internal fixation of the epiphysiolysis, with traction or plaster applied to the other fracture. In turn, type D fractures (one open fracture) are subjected to débridement and external fixation of the open fracture, with traction in the case of the closed fracture. Lastly, in type E fractures (open fractures of both bones), the authors perform external fixation of the tibial fracture and traction or external fixation of the femoral fracture. According to Letts et al., at least one of the two fractures should be rigidly fixed, the tibial fracture being the most appropriate candidate in most cases.

The authors also emphasized the age of the patients. In older children, intramedullary nailing of the femur and tibia may be more suitable than plate fixation. In children under 6 years of

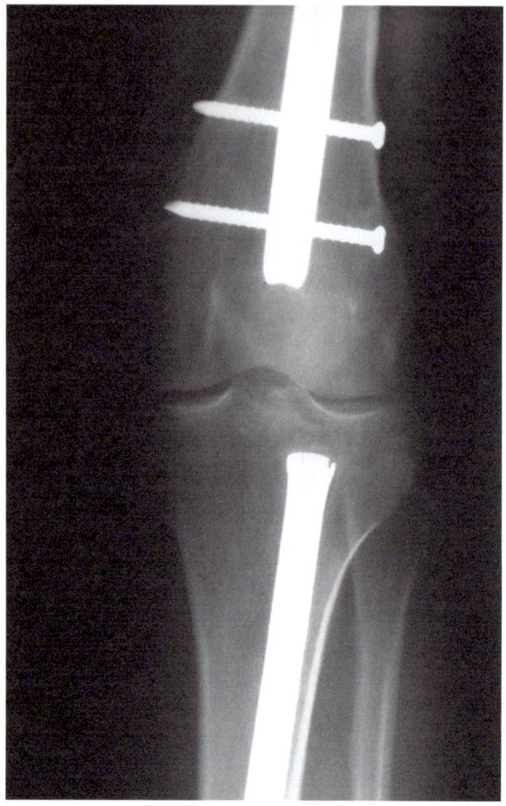

Fig 6.4 Anterograde nailing of both fractures (femoral and tibial) in another case of floating knee

age, stable closed reduction of the tibia can be achieved and maintained with a cast, while the femur is kept under traction. Surgical treatment of both fractures was not recommended, since this could give rise to overgrowth of the fractured extremity.

In 1991, Bohn and Durbin reviewed a series of 44 children and recommended conservative management of both fractures in patients under 10 years of age [6]. The indications of surgery for femoral fracture are serious head injuries, adolescents, significant soft tissue damage, and the impossibility of achieving adequate reduction through closed methods.

Yue et al. were not in agreement with these recommendations [18], however, since in their series of 30 patients followed-up for an average of 8.6 years, fewer complications (leg length discrepancies, delayed union, or deformities) and a shorter hospital stay were recorded in the patients subjected to surgery of both fractures, despite the fact that these individuals presented a poorer condition upon admission, as reflected by a poorer ISS score. These authors advised rigid stabilization at least of the femoral fracture, and preferably of both fractures, in patients belonging to any age group.

6.7 Results

In 1977, Karlstrom and Olerud established the criteria for assessing the results of treatment, and which subsequently have been adopted by the rest of the authors [24]. This classification evaluates symptoms from the thigh and leg, from the knee and ankle, walking stability, patient return to work and sports activities, deformity, shortening, and restricted joint mobility. Each of these parameters in turn is scored as excellent, good, acceptable, or poor. The presence of a single poor outcome corresponding to any of these parameters implies a poor overall outcome. In their series there were 16 excellent or good outcomes (59 %),

7 acceptable outcomes (26 %), and four poor outcomes (15 %).

Type II floating knees (with intraarticular involvement) often present poorer results than type I fractures. The severity of this fracture pattern was demonstrated in the series published by Adamson et al., who reviewed a total of 34 floating knee cases with involvement of the joint [10]. In one of our own series we recorded a high incidence of open fractures (62 %) and of vascular injuries (21 %), and 9 % of the patients suffered supracondylar amputation [25]. The mean postoperative range of movement was 96°, and 76 % of patients presented acceptable or poor results. We found type II floating knees to have a much poorer prognosis than type I fractures, and the results, moreover, were poorer than in other series. After reviewing 15 cases, we documented 5 good outcomes, 4 acceptable outcomes, and 6 poor outcomes. This was explained by the severity of the cases (with 10 open fractures, 6 cases of neurological damage, and 2 cases of vascular injury), as well as by the delay in definitive treatment (more than 12 days for the femoral fracture and up to 17 days in the case of the tibial fracture). Other studies carried out in our setting have reported good or excellent results in 54–63 % of cases [26, 27].

6.8 Complications

The severity of this range of injuries is reflected by the high frequency of complications. The largest series published to date reports 104 complications among 419 patients (24.8 %), and many of these complications were serious [2]. Chronic pain and knee stiffness are common in this kind of fractures. According to the literature, the mean range of movement varies from 92° [8] to 131° [9]. Early mobilization may help reduce the incidence of such problems. In many series, close to one-half of all patients suffer residual chronic knee pain [9, 25].

These individuals often require numerous reinterventions. In some cases the latter may comprise minor surgery, such as dynamization of a nail or implant removal, but in other cases major surgery is needed in the form of operations for infection or nonunions, for example, and which may imply the need for flaps, revascularization, grafting, and the replacement of osteosynthesis material.

Adamson et al. reported a 32 % infection rate in their series of 34 patients [10]. In the 11 cases of infection, the results were poor in 10 and acceptable in a single case, with the performance of three amputations. The amputation rate has been as high as 24 % in the series published by Paul et al. [8]. Most amputations are the result of catastrophic trauma with severe open fractures often associated to arterial damage.

Complications such as delayed union, nonunion, malunion, and joint stiffness are more frequent in patients with fractures of this kind than in individuals with isolated femoral or tibial fractures. Prolonged hospital stay is common, with a high risk of permanent disability and a high economic cost for society.

The infection rates vary greatly from one series to another. Fraser et al. reported a 30 % infection rate—this being the highest rate in all the known series to date [4]. Kao et al. in turn reported an infection rate of 20.8 % [2], while other authors have published figures of between 7 and 10 % [9, 24].

Pediatric patients in turn are characterized by a specific series of complications such as length discrepancies or genu valgum. Approximately one-third of all patients can present limb length discrepancy, either as a result of delayed growth (secondary to traumatic epiphysiodesis) or due to hyper growth reactive to the hyperemia caused by the fracture and by the surgical trauma [6]. Accordingly, shortening of 2–3 cm can be accepted in pediatric patients with diaphyseal fractures, since this length can be expected to be recovered over time.

6.9 Conclusions

The different variants of floating knee require individualized consideration of the type of fracture and of the general soft tissue conditions of the affected extremity. Regardless of the fixation technique used, an optimum outcome following intraarticular fracture depends on early mobilization and protected loading. The low incidence of floating knee, the heterogeneity of the fractures involved, and the different surgical techniques described in the literature complicate the definition of treatment strategies. However, based on the literature, we can recommend the surgical treatment of both fractures, except in non-displaced and stable fractures, where combined treatment could be considered (surgery for one of the fractures and conservative management for the other). In diaphyseal fractures it is advisable to perform intramedullary nailing (anterograde or retrograde, with or without reaming), depending on the characteristics of the fracture and the preferences of the surgeon. Non-displaced intraarticular fractures should be treated by percutaneous fixation and early mobilization. These lesions have fewer complications than displaced intraarticular fractures, which require anatomical reduction and internal fixation. The early loading recommended for diaphyseal fractures should be postponed if the patient has an ipsilateral intraarticular fracture. We usually first stabilize the femoral fracture, since it is normally a more severe fracture, with greater bleeding and a greater risk of fatal complications such as fat embolism. Fixation first of the femoral fracture avoids the risk of secondary femoral fracture displacement that could occur if tibial fracture stabilization were performed first. Manual traction without large angulations is required in order to avoid displacements of the tibial fracture during femoral fracture reduction. After fixation of the femoral fracture the knee can be flexed to secure a better access for insertion of a tibial nail. In floating knees with an open tibial fracture, the wound must be correctly irrigated and debrided before surgical stabilization of the femoral fracture. The tibial fracture can be stabilized using external fixation in order to reduce additional soft tissue damage during manipulation of the femoral fracture. Such fixation can be replaced by nailing or can be maintained as definitive treatment, depending on the severity of the soft tissue damage. After surgical stabilization of the femoral and tibial fractures, and provided the patient condition is acceptable, evaluation of the stability of the knee is indicated in order to diagnose possible ligament damage. Imaging studies should be performed as soon as possible to confirm such damage, though magnetic resonance imaging may be difficult to interpret in the presence of osteosynthesis material with a composition other than titanium. Medial collateral ligament damage is to be treated conservatively with an orthosis during 6 weeks. Damage to the lateral collateral ligament and posterolateral angle requires reconstruction in the early postoperative period, but not during stabilization of the fractures. Meniscal damage likewise should be resected and repaired during the early postoperative period, provided such damage produces symptoms. Cruciate ligament damage in turn requires deferred reconstruction.

References

1. Blake R, McBryde A Jr (1975) The floating knee: ipsilateral fractures of the tibia and femur. South Med J 68:13–16
2. Kao FC, Tu YK, Hsu KY, Su JY, Yen CY, Chou MC (2010) Floating knee injuries: a high complication rate. Orthopedics 33:14–19
3. Lundy DW, Johnson KD (2001) "Floating knee" injuries: ipsilateral fractures of the femur and tibia. J Am Acad Orthop Surg 9:238–245
4. Fraser RD, Hunter GA, Waddell JP (1978) Ipsilateral fracture of the femur and tibia. J Bone Joint Surg Br 60:510–515
5. Letts M, Vincent N, Gouw G (1986) The "floating knee" in children. J Bone Joint Surg Br 68:442–446
6. Bohn WW, Durbin RA (1991) Ipsilateral fractures of the femur and tibia in children and adolescents. J Bone Joint Surg Am 73:429–439
7. Arslan H, Kapukaya A, Kesemenli C, Subasi M, Kayikci C (2003) Floating knee in children. J Pediatr Orthop 23:458–463
8. Paul GR, Sawka MW, Whitelaw GP (1990) Fractures of the ipsilateral femur and tibia: emphasis on intra-articular and soft tissue injury. J Orthop Trauma 4:309–314
9. Veith RG, Winquist RA, Hansen ST Jr (1984) Ipsilateral fractures of the femur and tibia. A report of fifty-seven consecutive cases. J Bone Joint Surg Am 66:991–1002

10. Adamson GJ, Wiss DA, Lowery GL, Peters CL (1992) Type II floating knee: ipsilateral femoral and tibial fractures with intraarticular extension into the knee joint. J Orthop Trauma 6:333–339
11. Szalay MJ, Hosking OR, Annear P (1990) Injury of knee ligament associated with ipsilateral femoral shaft fractures and with ipsilateral femoral and tibial shaft fractures. Injury 21:398–400
12. Schiedts D, Mukisi M, Bouger D, Bastaraud H (1996) Ipsilateral fractures of the femoral and tibial diaphyses. Rev Chir Orthop Reparatrice Appar Mot 82:535–540
13. van Raay JJ, Raaymakers EL, Dupree HW (1991) Knee ligament injuries combined with ipsilateral tibial and femoral diaphyseal fractures: the "floating knee". Arch Orthop Trauma Surg 110:75–77
14. Pape HC, Giannoudis P, Krettek C (2002) The timing of fracture treatment in polytrauma patients: relevance of damage control orthopedic surgery. Am J Surg 183:622–629
15. Hee HT, Wong HP, Low YP, Myers L (2001) Predictors of outcome of floating knee injuries in adults: 89 patients followed for 2–12 years. Acta Orthop Scand 72:385–394
16. Hung SH, Lu YM, Huang HT, Lin YK, Chang JK, Chen JC, Tien YC, Huang PJ, Chen CH, Liu PC, Chao D (2007) Surgical treatment of type II floating knee: comparisons of the results of type IIA and type IB floating knee. Knee Surg Sports Traumatol Arthrosc 15:578–586
17. Dwyer AJ, Paul R, Mam MK, Kumar A, Gosselin RA (2005) Floating knee injuries: long-term results of four treatment methods. Int Orthop 29:314–318
18. Yue JJ, Churchill RS, Cooperman DR, Yasko AW, Wilber JH, Thompson GH (2000) The floating knee in the pediatric patient. Nonoperative versus operative stabilization. Clin Orthop Relat Res 376:124–136
19. Rooser B, Hansson P (1985) External fixation of ipsilateral fractures of the femur and tibia. Injury 16:371–373
20. Behr JT, Apel DM, Pinzur MS, Dobozi WR, Behr MJ (1987) Flexible intramedullary nails for ipsilateral femoral and tibial fractures. J Trauma 27:1354–1357
21. Gregory P, DiCicco J, Karpik K, DiPasquale T, Herscovici D, Sanders R (1996) Ipsilateral fractures of the femur and tibia: treatment with retrograde femoral nailing and unreamed tibial nailing. J Orthop Trauma 10:309–316
22. Ostrum RF (2000) Treatment of floating knee injuries through a single percutaneous approach. Clin Orthop Relat Res 375:43–50
23. Rethnam U (2006) Single incision nailing of the floating knee: do we ignore the knee ligaments? Int Orthop 30:311–317
24. Karlstrom G, Olerud S (1997) Ipsilateral fracture of the femur and tibia. J Bone Joint Surg Am 59:240–243
25. Oñorbe F, Ferrer-Santacreu EM, Rodríguez-Merchán EC (2008) Rodilla flotante: revision retrospectiva de 15 casos tratados durante un periodo de 5 años. Rev Ortop Traumatol 52:283–289
26. Ríos A, Fahandezh-Saddi H, Martín-García A, Martínez-Gómiz JM, Villa A, Vaquero J (2003) Rodilla flotante traumatica: A propósito de 21 casos. Rev Ortop Traumatol 47:311–316
27. Miralles-Muñoz FA, Lizaúr-Utrilla A, Bustamante-Suárez D (2005) La rodilla flotante: studio retrospective de 41 casos. Rev Ortop Traumatol 49:255–259

Nonunion and Malunion Around the Knee

7

Juan Carlos Rubio-Suárez

7.1 Introduction

Current techniques and recent osteosynthesis implant designs along with greater care of soft tissue provide excellent results in the treatment of fractures around the knee, with union rates near 100 % in some cases [1–3].

However, some authors have published rates of nonunion in 9 % of cases in distal femoral fractures and 4 % in proximal tibial fractures [4, 5]. The nonunion is more frequent in the metaphyseal segment of the fracture, while intraarticular nonunions are uncommon [6].

The incidence of reported malunion is 42 % in distal femoral fractures and 31 % in proximal tibial fractures (79 % in patients over 60 years) [7]. Most malunion show malalignment due to alteration of the mechanical axis that increases the likelihood of developing osteoarthritis in the knee joint. Rotational deformities are less common and require CT scan study for diagnostic [8].

7.2 Etiology

Nonunions and malunion are caused by multiple etiological factors such as:

- Comorbidities: diabetes or other metabolic diseases, vascular insufficiency, prior or concomitant infections, obesity, treatment with NSAIDs, and smoker patients.
- Type of fracture: high comminution, open fracture, and severe damage to the soft tissues.
- Osteosynthesis: poor indication or poor surgical technique, lack of grafting, poor reduction.
- Postoperative care: too early weight bearing of the affected limb, unruly patient, poor or no rehabilitation.

7.3 Evaluation

A good clinical history is paramount to collect all data related to the patient, to the fracture, and also to the treatment and its evolution.

Then, a good physical examination is mandatory, with special attention to:

- Soft tissues: scars, fistulas, drains, erythema.
- Vascular status of the lower limbs.
- Knee range of motion as well as ipsilateral hip and ankle mobility.
- Limb alignment and rotation compared with the contralateral side.
- Length of the lower limbs.

7.3.1 Radiological Examination

- Simple anterior–posterior and lateral views of the knee. Sometimes oblique views can be useful.

J. C. Rubio-Suárez (✉)
Department of Orthopaedic Surgery, "La Paz" University Hospital-IdiPaz, Paseo de la Castellana, 261, Madrid, 28046, Spain
e-mail: rubioj57@gmail.com

E. C. Rodríguez-Merchán (ed.), *Traumatic Injuries of the Knee*,
DOI: 10.1007/978-88-470-5298-7_7, © Springer-Verlag Italia 2013

- Long-standing X-rays of the lower limbs: will provide information about potential malalignment and/or leg length discrepancy.
- Computed tomography (CT) scan: is useful in detecting changes in the rotation of the affected limb.

7.3.2 Laboratory Tests

- Routine blood test.
- Serological test to detect infection: ESR (erythrocyte sedimentation rate) and CRP (C-reactive protein).
- Exudation culture in case of suppuration.

7.4 Treatment

7.4.1 Nonsurgical Treatment

Most cases require surgical management. Nonsurgical treatment would be indicated in those patients unable to walk but without pain and also in patients with comorbidities (high surgical risk). An orthosis to control instability along with physical therapy (ultrasounds, shock waves, electro stimulation) can be successful in these patients.

7.4.2 Surgical Treatment

Preoperative planning is mandatory. We must make the appropriate measurements on radiographic imaging to determine the corrections that we are going to perform. In addition, we can anticipate the implants that we are going to need and the surgical approach that will be necessary. It is also important to plan surgical approaches and if necessary we will need the help of a plastic surgeon. In summary, this type of surgery is complex enough to go to the operating room with everything perfectly planned.

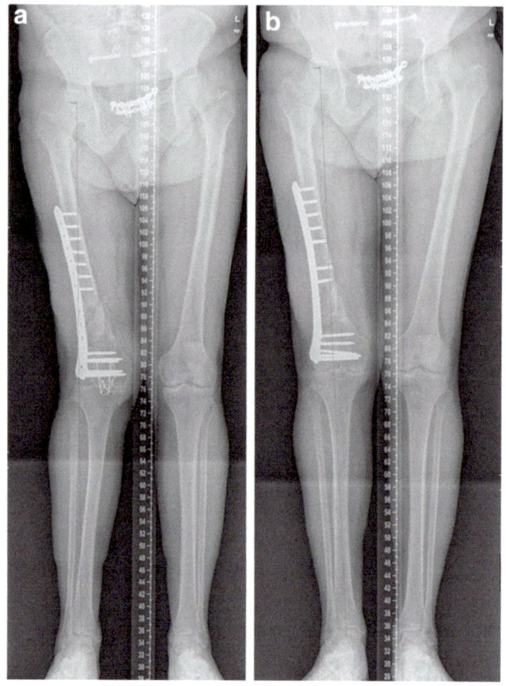

Fig. 7.1 (**a**) Distal femoral fracture in polytrauma patient. Open reduction and internal fixation (ORIF) with a locking compression plate: valgus of the right knee (malunion) after the first surgical procedure; (**b**) correct alignment after revision of the previous ORIF

Open Reduction and Internal Fixation (ORIF)

It is the treatment of choice and leads to good results in 95 % of the cases [9]. The ORIF indications are: young patients with a good range of knee mobility, good condition of the articular cartilage, bone stock enough, and good soft tissues. In contrast, ORIF would not be indicated in cases of bone loss, hardware remaining, knee stiffness, or bone dystrophy.

No implant has proved to be better than another. However, there is agreement that locked plates with angular stability provide excellent results in most cases [10] (Fig. 7.1).

Intramedullary nailing is also a good tool for treatment. It is a minimally invasive method that respects the soft tissues and has excellent mechanical properties because it is located in the

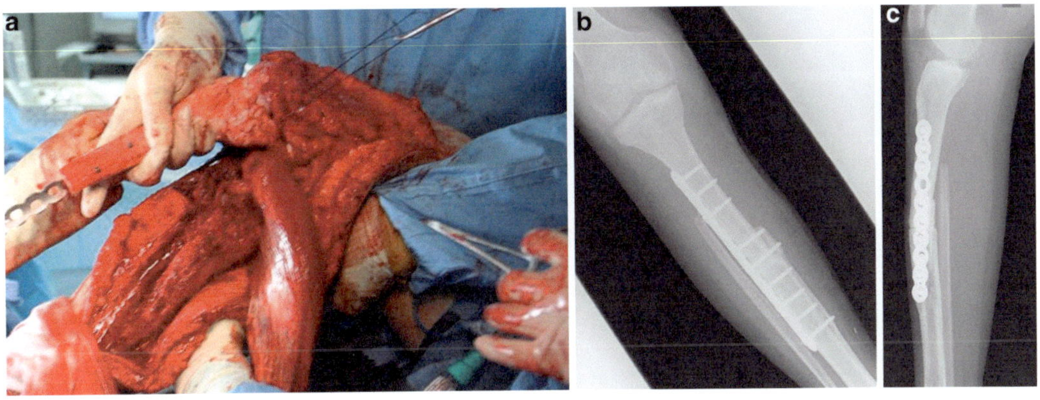

Fig. 7.2 Fresh frozen allograft in the treatment of a nonunion of a complex proximal tibial fracture: (**a**) intraoperative image; (**b**) postoperative AP view; (**c**) postoperative lateral view

load axis. However, when the epiphyseal segment is too short (<4 cm) the intramedullary nail does not provide adequate fixation. In these cases, failure occurs in 33.3 % [11]. This could be avoided with new designs of nails.

ORIF should be accompanied by bone graft. Autologous graft is the most used. Osteoconductive and osteoinductive substances have been used with more or less success. Biological substances such as bone morphogenetic protein (BMP) and platelet growth factor (PGF) are expensive and have been used in the last years with poor results [12], [13]. Nowadays, pluripotential stem cells from bone marrow or adipose tissue are being researched with encouraging results [14].

Nevertheless, the ORIF in nonunions and malunion presents a high rate of complications such as knee stiffness, malunion (>50 %), hardware intolerance, infection, and posttraumatic osteoarthritis.

External Fixation

External fixation is a valid alternative to ORIF. It is a minimal invasive method, so it is specially indicated in cases of nonunion with poor soft tissues. The most used at present are those devices that combine fine wires and circular rings, such as the hybrid AO-ASIF external fixator [15], the Ilizarov, and the Taylor spatial frame [16].

Published results are excellent, achieving union in most cases [15], [16]. However, the average fixator time in place was 310 days and knee stiffness occurred in 78 % [17].

External fixators are also indicated in cases of septic nonunions and large bone defects because they allow us to make a bone transport. The results have been successful but the learning curve is long. Moreover, the treatment is long and therefore the fixator time is also long, so it is poorly tolerated by the patient [18].

Allografts

Osteoarticular allografts are indicated in cases of great joint destruction with a lot of bone and cartilage loss, especially in active young patients. The published results with fresh frozen osteochondral allografts have been very good (Fig. 7.2). The survivorship at 5 years is 95 % and at 10 years it is 80–85 % [19]. However, the survivorship at 20 years is only 46 % and the surviving grafts showed a moderate to severe degree of osteoarthritis or collapse. Moreover, allografts can be a source of transmissible diseases and require a complex and expensive transplant program. In summary, osteoarticular allografts represent an alternative treatment for active young patients to delay as much as possible a total knee arthroplasty.

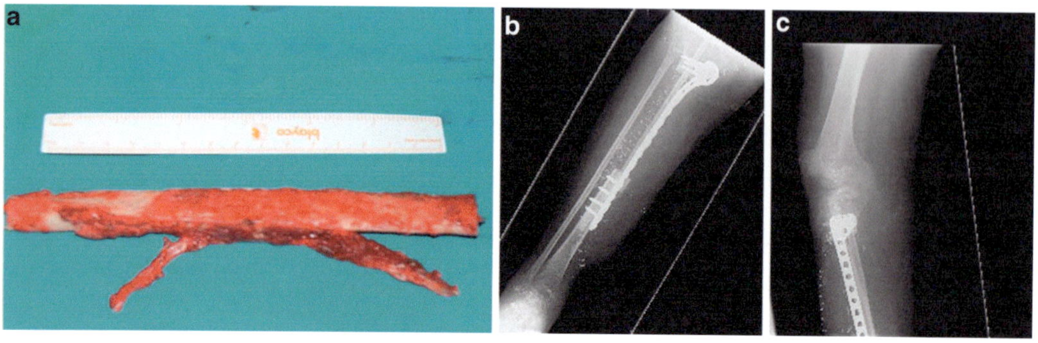

Fig. 7.3 Free fibular autograft in double bar to treat a great bone defect in a complex fracture of the proximal tibia: (**a**) intraoperative view of the fibular graft; (**b**) postoperative AP view; (**c**) postoperative lateral view

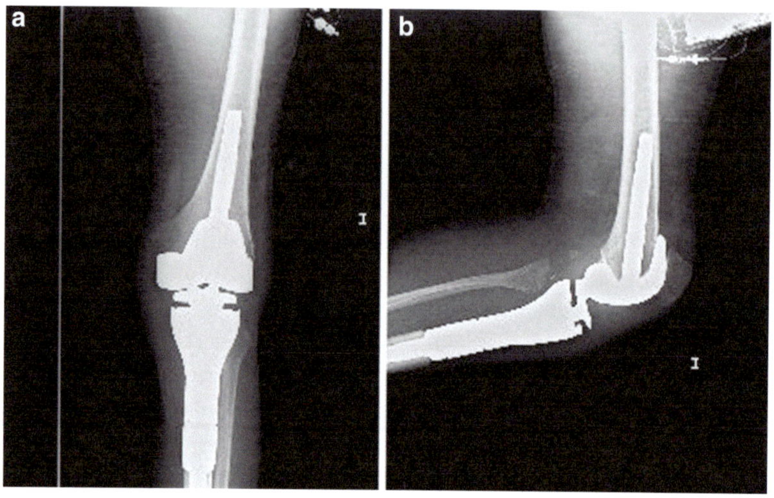

Fig. 7.4 Tumoral megaprosthesis to treat a complex intraarticular proximal tibial fracture: (**a**) AP postoperative view; (**b**) postoperative lateral view

Free Autografts

Vascularized autografts are indicated in cases such as:

- Great bone loss but no affectation of articular surface.
- Poor soft tissues state after great traumatisms and open fractures.
- Chronic infection.
- Post-irradiation.

The most extended graft is the fibular middle shaft which allows us to get a bone segment 20 cm long or more. The fibular segment can be used as a single or double bar (Fig. 7.3). Published results of fibular graft show high success rates [20]. However, free fibular bone graft may have disadvantages such as residual limb differences, stress fractures, and is technically demanding. Hence it is not a method that can be routinely used.

Total Joint Arthroplasty

It is indicated in severe posttraumatic osteoarthritis in patients over 60-years old. It allows the patient an immediate weight bearing and a good range of knee motion and pain relief [21].

Total knee arthroplasty requires a long and complex surgery with large soft tissue releases, hardware removing, and ligament repair in one surgical stage. We can use any implant design but most authors recommend constrained designs, revision designs with femoral and tibial stems, including tumoral mega prosthesis in cases of great bone loss (Fig. 7.4). When malalignment exists we recommend computer assisted surgery.

The complications rate of this treatment is high (29–47 %). More common complications are instability, stiffness, chronic pain, infection, and soft tissue damage [21, 22].

Arthrodesis (Joint Fusion)

Its main use is as a salvage of failed arthroplasty. However, it is also used in severe infection, extensor mechanism deficiency, or massive bone loss. In contrast, we must not perform an arthrodesis in cases of ipsilateral hip fusion or contralateral knee fusion.

Knee arthrodesis can be performed in different ways such as external fixation, plate and screws, or intramedullary nailing. There are no differences in the results, but the use of autologous bone graft to refill the defect is recommended [23]. Special care must be taken to leave the knee in 5–7 of valgus and 10–15 of flexion.

Persistent pain, back pain, and patient cosmetic dissatisfaction are common complications. But the commonest one is the persistent nonunion due to poor surgical technique, infection, or a deficient bone stock [23].

7.5 Conclusions

Complications after fractures around the knee are becoming less frequent due to better osteosynthesis techniques, greater care of the soft tissues, and strict action protocols. The main complications are malunion and nonunion, and their treatment is difficult and highly demanding. Nonsurgical management is reserved for non-walking patients with no pain and high surgical risk.

In most cases, surgical treatment is indicated. Modern osteosynthesis plates with angular stability head screws are an excellent tool which provides good stability and allows early mobilization. Intramedullary nailing is indicated in supracondylar nonunions with good results, but its use is not recommended when the epiphyseal fragment is less than 4 cm. In cases of severe infection, great deformities or great bone defects, external fixation is the main indication. Devices such as Ilizarov or Taylor frame, using small wires and rings, are commonly used.

Allografts have a half-life of no more than 15–20 years. Hence their main indication is a young active patient with great articular destruction. The goal is to provide him/her with a good quality of life and delay a total knee arthroplasty.

The arthroplasty aims to relieve pain and provide good function. It is indicated in patients over 60 years and constrained or revision devices are recommended in all cases. In cases with severe bone loss, tumoral megaprostheses are indicated.

Joint fusion (arthrodesis)is the salvage method in cases of arthroplasty failure or non-controlled severe infection. It is not indicated when ipsilateral hip or contralateral knee is fused.

Whatever the chosen method of treatment, it should be preceded by good preoperative planning.

References

1. Kregor PJ, Stannard JA, Zlowodzki M, Cole PA (2004) Treatment of distal femur fractures using the less invasive stabilization system: surgical experience and early clinical results in 103 fractures. J Orthop Trauma 18:509–520
2. Ricci AR, Yue JJ, Taffet R, Catalano JB, DeFalco RA, Wilkens KJ (2004) Less invasive stabilization system for treatment of distal femur fractures. Am J Orthop 33:250–255
3. Weight M, Collinge C (2004) Early results of the less invasive stabilization system for mechanically unstable fractures of the distal femur. J Orthop Trauma 18:503–508
4. Graves ML, Ryan JE, Mast JW (2005) Supracondylar femur non-union associated with previous vascular repair: importance of vascular exam in preoperative planning of non-union repair. J Orthop Trauma 19:574–577
5. Papagelopoulos PJ, Partsinevelos AA, Themistocleous GS, Mavrogenis AF, Korres DS, Soucacos PN (2006) Complications after tibia plateau fracture surgery. Injury. 37:475–484
6. King GJ, Schatzker J (1991) Non-union of a complex tibial plateau fracture. J Orthop Trauma 5:209–212
7. Davison BL (2003) Varus collapse of comminuted distal femur fractures after open reduction and internal fixation with a lateral condylar buttress plate. Am J Orthop 32:27–30
8. Rosen AL, Strauss E (2004) Primary total knee arthroplasty for complex distal femur fractures in elderly patients. Clin Orthop Relat Res 425:101–105

9. Haidukewych GJ, Berry DJ, Jacofsky DJ, Torchia ME (2003) Treatment of supracondylar femur nonunions with open reduction and internal fixation. Am J Orthop 32:564–567
10. Hailer YD, Hoffman R (2006) Management of nonunion of the distal femur in osteoporotic bone with the internal fixation system LISS. Arch Orthop Trauma Surg 126:350–353
11. Wu CC, Shih CH (1991) Distal femoral non-union treated with interlocking nailing. J Trauma 31:1659–1662
12. Butcher A, Milner R, Keith E et al (2009) Interaction of platelet-rich concentrate with bone graft materials: an in vitro study. J Orthop Trauma 23:195–202
13. Parsons P, Butcher A, Hesselden K et al (2008) Platelet-rich concentrate supports human mesenchymal stem cell proliferation, bone morphogenetic protein-2 messenger RNA expression, alkaline phosphatase activity, and bone formation in vitro: A mode of action to enhance bone repair. J Orthop Trauma 22:595–604
14. Thomas SO, David Y, Kristen L et al (2012) Mesenchymal stem cells facilitate fracture repair in an alcohol-induced impaired healing model. J Orthop Trauma 26:712–718
15. Lonner JH, Siliski JM, Jupiter JB, Lhowe DW (1999) Posttraumatic non-union of the proximal tibial metaphysis. Am J Orthop 28:523–528
16. Feldman DS, Shin SS, Madan S, Koval K (2003) Correction of tibial malunion and non-union with six-axis analysis deformity correction using the Taylor Spatial Frame. J Orthop Trauma 17:549–554
17. Saridis A, Panagiotopoulos E, Tyllianakis M, Matzaroglou C, Vandoros N, Lambiris E (2006) The use of the Ilizarov method as a salvage procedure in infected non-union of the distal femur with bone loss. J Bone Joint Surg Br 88:232–237
18. Bellabarba C, Ricci WM, Bolhofner BR (2002) Indirect reduction and plating of distal femoral nonunions. J Orthop Trauma 16:287–296
19. Gross AE, Shasha N, Aubin P (2005) Long-term followup of the use of fresh osteochondral allografts for posttraumatic knee defects. Clin Orthop Relat Res 435:79–87
20. Muramatsu K, Ihara K, Shigetomi M, Kawai S (2004) Femoral reconstruction by single, folded or double free vascularised fibular grafts. Br J Plast Surg 57:550–555
21. Haidukewych GJ, Springer BD, Jacofsky DJ, Berry DJ (2005) Total knee arthroplasty for salvage of failed internal fixation of non-union of the distal femur. J Arthroplasty 20:344–349
22. Wu L, Xiong Y, Yan S, Yang OS (2005) Total knee replacement for posttraumatic degenerative arthritis of the knee. Chinese J Traumatol. 8:195–199
23. Figgie HE III, Brody GA, Inglis AE, Sculco TP, Goldberg VM, Figgie MP (1987) Knee arthrodesis following total knee arthroplasty in rheumatoid arthritis. Clin Orthop Relat Res 224:237–243

8 Knee Extensor Mechanism Injuries

Fares S. Haddad and Senthooran Raja

8.1 Introduction

The extensor mechanism of the knee consists of the quadriceps muscle complex, quadriceps tendon, patella, patellar tendon and its insertion onto the tibial tubercle [1].

The principle function of the extensor mechanism of the knee is to maintain an erect position [2]. Its ability to overcome gravity is demonstrated through ambulation, standing from a seated position and walking up and down stairs. Injury to the extensor mechanism can be potentially devastating to everyday life.

Divergent forces generated by the contraction of the quadriceps femoris converge via the patella and patellar tendon onto the tibial tubercle and result in active knee extension [3]. The patella acts as a fulcrum and its main biomechanical function is to improve quadriceps efficiency by increasing the lever arm of the extensor mechanism [4]. The patella does this in two ways; first, by linking the quadriceps tendon with the patellar tendon and second, by displacing the tendon linkage away from the axis of knee rotation. This increases the lever arm as the knee extends and provides the extra torque required to achieve the terminal 15° of active knee extension [2].

F. S. Haddad (✉) · S. Raja
University College London Hospital NHS Trust, Euston Road, London, NW12BU, UK
e-mail: fsh@fareshaddad.net

Injury to the extensor mechanism usually occurs as a result of indirect trauma excluding patellar fractures [1, 5].

Injuries may occur at any level in the extensor mechanism and are described here in further detail.

8.2 Quadriceps Tendon Rupture

8.2.1 Epidemiology

Quadriceps tendon rupture is uncommon, accounting for 3 % of all tendon injuries [6]. It tends to occur in those over the age of 40 years with a peak incidence in the sixth and seventh decades of life. A strong male pre-ponderance exists, many authors reporting men being eight times more likely to sustain a unilateral quadriceps tendon rupture when compared to women.

The non-dominant limb is affected in twice as many cases as the dominant limb [7]. Bilateral simultaneous quadriceps tendon rupture is a rare entity and tends to occur in patients with predisposing medical conditions [8].

8.2.2 Aetiology

Forced, rapid contraction of the quadriceps muscle in a partially flexed knee is the typical mechanism of injury in acute quadriceps tendon rupture.

E. C. Rodríguez-Merchán (ed.), *Traumatic Injuries of the Knee*,
DOI: 10.1007/978-88-470-5298-7_8, © Springer-Verlag Italia 2013

Risk factors include chronic renal failure, diabetes mellitus, hyperparathyroidism, gout, obesity and either local or systemic corticosteroids use [9]. Repetitive microtrauma and subsequent degeneration of the tendon reduces tensile strength thus pre-disposing to rupture [6].

8.2.3 Anatomy

The quadriceps tendon has a trilaminar arrangement. The most superficial layer being derived from the rectus femoris tendon, the middle layer is formed by vastus lateralis and vastus medialis. Finally, vastus intermedius provides the deep layer of the quadriceps tendon [10].

The medial and lateral patellar retinacula are formed predominantly by the fibres of the vastus medialis and lateralis respectively [2]. The lateral retinaculum also receives fibres from the iliotibial tract [8]. These act as the auxilary extensors of the knee, hence preserving some degree of active extension in quadriceps tendon ruptures [9].

Ruptures frequently begin in the rectus femoris tendon extending into the vastus intermedius or move transversely to either medial or lateral patellar retinaculum. Ruptures in the elderly arise at the osteotendinous junction within 3 cms proximal of the superior pole of the patella [11]. Ruptures within the midsubstance of the tendon or musculotendinous region are infrequent and are commoner in young adults [8].

8.2.4 Diagnosis

Early diagnosis is essential in acute quadriceps tendon rupture as delayed surgical repair is associated with adverse outcomes [12].

The triad of acute knee pain, palpable suprapatellar gap and loss of active extension is pathognomonic of acute quadriceps tendon rupture [3, 8]. Unfortunately, this injury may be accompanied by a large haemarthrosis which obscures clinical findings.

As mentioned previously, the patellar retinaculum acts as an auxiliary extensor of the knee. Hence it is important to distinguish between full and weak active knee extension. In the absence of active knee extension a complete quadriceps tendon rupture and patellar retinaculum is probable. If the patellar retinaculum remains intact, weak extension might be elicited. Partial ruptures may present with a palpable suprapatellar defect but full active knee extension [2].

Although diagnosis is clinical, radiographs contribute evidence of an acute rupture [13]. Positive findings on a lateral radiograph (with the injured knee flexed to 30°) include obliteration of the quadriceps tendon shadow, suprapatellar mass and an inferiorly displaced patella (baja) [14] (Fig. 8.1).

Blumensaat's line and the Insall-Salvati ratio are both methods of evaluating the patellar height on a lateral radiograph [15] (Fig. 8.2).

Blumensaat's line is a straight line drawn along the opacity given by the intercondylar notch of the distal femur. The inferior pole of the patella usually rests on this line. The lower pole of the patella will lie inferior (patella baja) to this line in quadriceps tendon rupture or superiorly (patella alta) in cases of patellar tendon rupture.

The Insall-Salvati method indirectly assesses patellar height using a ratio of the length of the patellar tendon to the length of the patella [16]. The T/P ratio should range from 0.8 to 1.2. If it is greater than 1.2 it is considered patella alta and may support a diagnosis of patellar tendon rupture. In patella baja the T/P ratio will be less than 0.8, suggesting quadriceps tendon rupture.

The role of MRI and ultrasound is useful in unclear diagnoses. Ultrasound provides a cheap and readily available diagnostic tool, but is operator dependent [3, 4]. MRI is the gold standard investigation, but due to its lack of availability in many hospitals and clinics it may delay diagnosis [17].

8.2.5 Management

Incomplete rupture of the quadriceps tendon may be treated non-operatively [2, 3, 7, 9]. This involves cylinder cast or brace immobilisation in full extension for a minimum of 4–6 weeks,

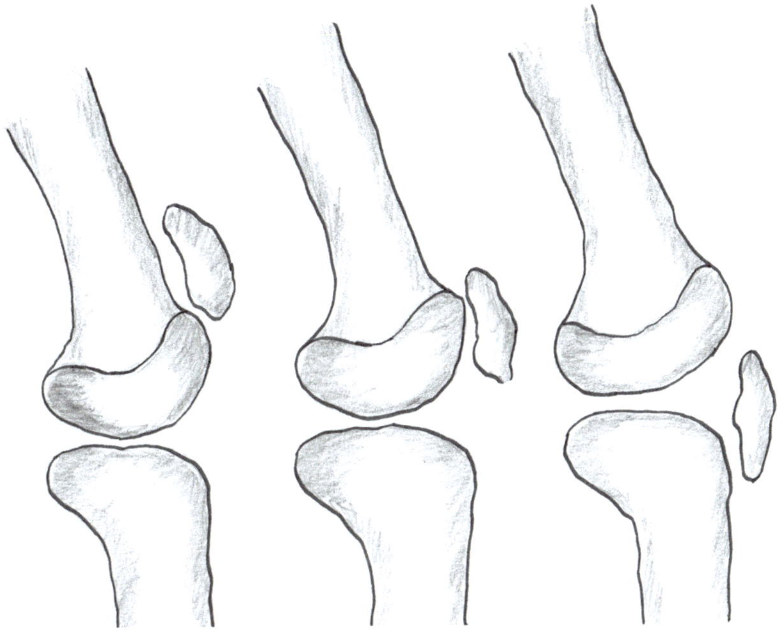

Fig. 8.1 Although diagnosis of an acute quadriceps tendon rupture is clinical, radiographs contribute evidence. Positive findings on a lateral radiograph (with the injured knee flexed to 30°) include obliteration of the quadriceps tendon shadow, suprapatellar mass and an inferiorly displaced patella (baja)

followed by physiotherapy geared towards promoting knee flexion and increasing quadriceps strength [5, 9].

Complete ruptures require urgent primary surgical repair as soon as they are diagnosed [18, 19]. If surgery is delayed, the tendon retracts proximally and binds down to the femur, making surgical repair difficult and functional outcomes poor [2, 18].

A tear at the musculotendinous junction or midsubstance requires end-to-end primary repair [3, 5, 12].

Osteotendinous quadriceps tendon ruptures are treated with transosseous sutures tied at the distal pole of the patella (Fig. 8.3).

A midline incision is used to expose the tendon rupture and patella. The tear is then elevated medially and laterally to reveal the apex of any patellar retinaculum tear if present [3]. These are sutured but left untied until the tendon repair is complete.

Heavy, non-absorbable sutures (e.g. Ethibond® 3) are placed in the proximal tendon remnant with a locking technique such as those described by Kessler, Krakow or Bunnell [20]. The suture ends are then passed through the patella via pre-drilled parallel longitudinal bone tunnels and tied distally at the inferior pole of the patella [2, 5, 9, 12, 21].

Care must be taken to avoid too anterior an entry point into the patella as this may lead to patellar tilting. Other operative methods such as those using suture anchors, or a transverse bone tunnel have been described but no one technique has been shown to yield superior results over the other [22].

Most repairs are reinforced with a distally based partial thickness triangular flap of tendon, which is then reflected over the suture line, otherwise known as the Scuderi repair [3, 5].

Post-operatively, the knee is immobilised in full extension for 6 weeks followed by physiotherapy.

8.2.6 Complications

Most retrospective case series have shown good to excellent functional outcomes in complete unilateral quadriceps tendon ruptures treated surgically.

Timing of surgery is undecided, as some studies demonstrate good results after immediate repair, with others showing poor outcomes only

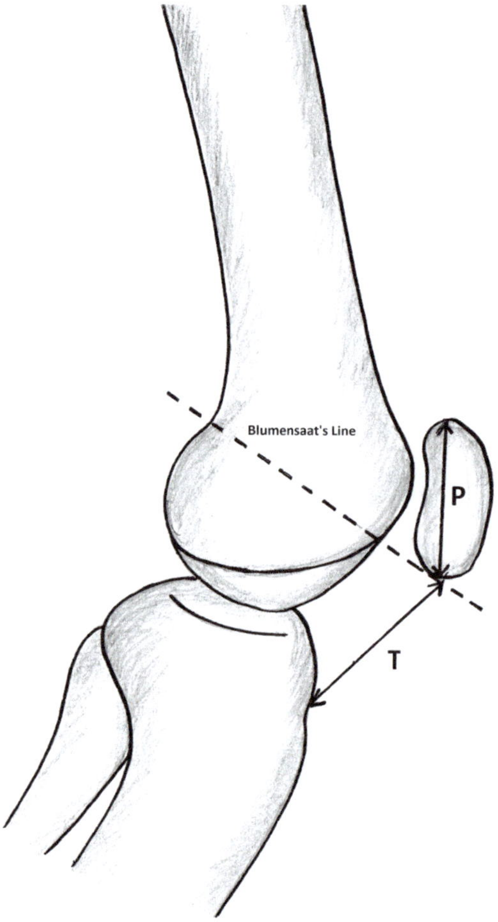

Fig. 8.2 Blumensaat's line and the Insall-Salvati ratio (T/P) are both methods of evaluating the patellar height on a lateral radiograph. The T/P ratio should range from 0.8 to 1.2. If it is greater than 1.2 it is considered patella alta and may support a diagnosis of patellar tendon rupture. In patella baja the T/P ratio will be less than 0.8, suggesting quadriceps tendon rupture. *P* length of patella. *T* Length of patellar tendon

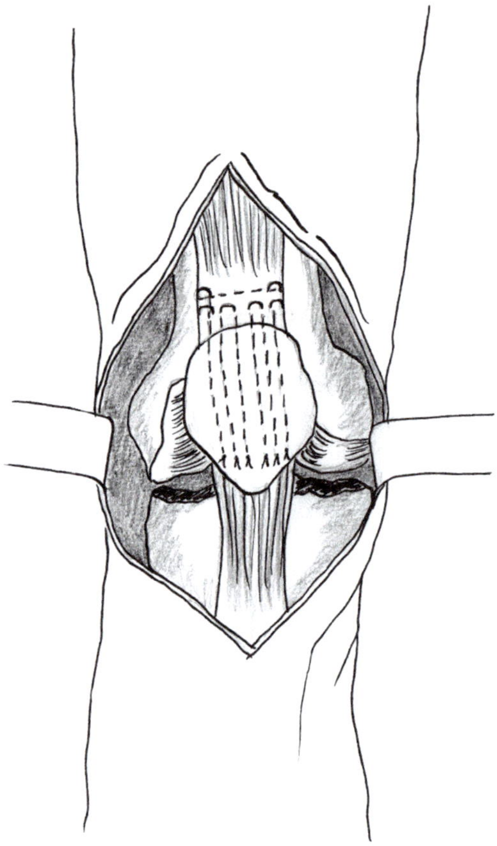

Fig. 8.3 Transosseous suture tied at the distal pole of the patella to treat an osteotendinous quadriceps tendon rupture. A midline incision is used to expose the tendon rupture and patella. The tear is then elevated medially and laterally to reveal the apex of any patellar retinaculum tear if present. These are sutured but left untied until the tendon repair is complete. Heavy, non-absorbable sutures (e.g. Ethibond® 3) are placed in the proximal tendon remnant with a locking technique. The suture ends are then passed through the patella via pre-drilled parallel longitudinal bone tunnels and tied distally at the inferior pole of the patella. Care must be taken to avoid too anterior an entry point into the patella as this may lead to patellar tilting

when surgery is delayed by more than 2 weeks [3, 18]. The general consensus is to repair acute ruptures as soon as they are diagnosed.

Although a healthy range of movement (0–120°) or more can be expected following prompt surgical repair, many individuals are unable to return to their usual recreational activities and up to 16 % are unable to return to work [5, 6, 19].

Complications include quadriceps atrophy or weakness, extensor lag, re-rupture, stiffness and diminished knee flexion [3, 6–9].

8.3 Patellar Tendon Rupture

8.3.1 Epidemiology

Patellar tendon ruptures are less common than quadriceps tendon ruptures [9, 23]. Eighty per cent occur in individuals aged less than 40-years old [24]. This injury is frequently described in athletes [25].

8.3.2 Aetiology

Much like quadriceps tendon ruptures, an indirect mechanism of injury is typically the cause.

Pre-existing patellar tendonitis and degenerative tendinosis are major risk factors for rupture [1, 5, 7, 24]. There is a lesser association with chronic disease states compared to quadriceps tendon rupture [25]. However, midsubstance patellar tendon tears are more likely to be associated with systemic disease.

8.3.3 Anatomy

The patellar tendon emerges from the inferior pole of the patella as a continuation of the quadriceps tendon. The majority of its fibres are received from the rectus femoris tendon and on average is 5 cm in length [2].

The patellar tendon is a strong, flat structure approximately 4–6 mm thick [2, 9]. The posterior aspect of the patellar tendon receives its blood supply from the inferomedial and inferolateral geniculate arteries via the infrapatellar fat pad [26]. The recurrent tibial and inferomedial geniculate arteries supply the anterior surface of the tendon [2, 9, 26].

The patellar tendon is relatively avascular at its proximal and distal ends making it susceptible to rupture at these sites [5, 9]. The commonest location for rupture is at the junction between tendon and the inferior pole of the patella [1, 5, 27].

8.3.4 Diagnosis

Acute ruptures are frequently missed [7]. They present with pain, swelling and bruising in and around the patella. An audible 'pop' may be heard and weight-bearing is difficult [1, 5].

Examination can reveal a palpable defect distal to the inferior pole of the patella and the patella migrated proximally due to unopposed quadriceps contraction [24].

Active knee extension against gravity is diminished or absent. If the patellar retinaculum is intact active extension may be possible, with or without an extensor lag [24].

Rupture typically presents as a final stage in degenerative tendinopathy and hence calcification may be visible on radiographs [9, 28]. A small bony fragment avulsed from the inferior pole of the patella at the time of rupture, might also be seen [5]. Patella alta should be observed for on lateral views as previously described.

USS has advantages over MRI, as it allows dynamic evaluation of the tendon and is cheaper and more accessible [29]. Both modalities can distinguish between partial and full thickness tears, however, MRI is better if suspecting intra-articular pathology [5, 9, 13, 28].

8.3.5 Management

A partial thickness tear in the presence of full active knee extension is treated non-operatively [1, 5, 9, 30].

Special consideration is given to athletes as the patellar tendon is exposed to repetitive eccentric loading [31]. There is a greater risk of complete rupture with conservative management and surgical intervention is associated with a return to premorbid sports activities [32, 33].

Earlier surgical repair of acute patellar tendon ruptures correlates with a better clinical outcome [9, 28]. Midsubstance tears once exposed through a midline incision are first debrided and reattached with a running interlocking non-absorbable stitch. For example, two Krakow locking stitches are placed in both proximal and distal ends of the ruptured tendon. The proximal and distal sutures are then tied together with the knee in full extension [30]. Retinaculum tears are primarily repaired using heavy absorbable sutures and the paratenon closed if possible [30, 34].

To alleviate tension on the suture line and protect the repair, a cerclage wire or cable can be placed through the patella and tibial tuberosity [5]. This allows for more aggressive post-operative rehabilitation. The wire or cable is removed after 6–8 weeks.

Acute ruptures arising at the bone–tendon junction utilise a transosseous fixation to restore continuity [24] (Fig. 8.4).

Adequate exposure of the patella and distal end of the tendon rupture is obtained through a midline incision. Flakes of bone avulsed from the patella should be excised and the edges of the ruptured tendon freshened [30]. Non-absorbable locking sutures are applied to the end of the ruptured patellar tendon and passed through longitudinal bone tunnels pre-drilled in the patella and tied proximally [1, 9, 25, 27, 34].

Important considerations include reattaching the tendon adjacent to the articular surface of the patella to prevent tilting and applying sufficient tension to the repair so no gaps appear when passively flexing the knee intraoperatively [9, 27].

Semitendinosus allograft or autografts may be employed to protect surgical repair as well as cerclage wire or cables, however, case series have shown excellent functional outcomes in repairs performed without augmentation [35, 36].

The knee is immobilised in full extension while weight bearing for 6 weeks [5, 24]. Post-operative rehabilitation is crucial in producing optimal functional outcomes.

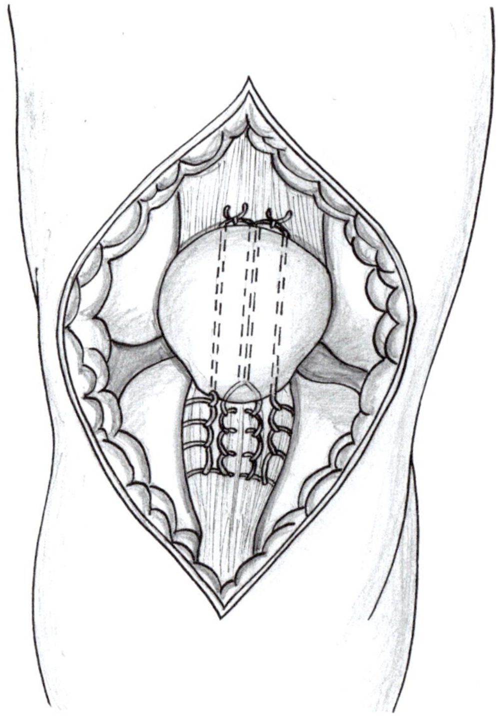

Fig. 8.4 Transosseous fixation of an acute rupture of the patellar tendon arising at the bone–tendon junction in order to restore continuity. Adequate exposure of the patella and distal end of the tendon rupture is obtained through a midline incision. Flakes of bone avulsed from the patella should be excised and the edges of the ruptured tendon freshened. Non-absorbable locking sutures are applied to the end of the ruptured patellar tendon and passed through longitudinal bone tunnels pre-drilled in the patella and tied proximally

The late reconstruction of the patellar tendon described by Ecker et al. uses a Steinmann pin inserted transversely through the patella to provide skeletal traction distally. The semitendinosus and gracilis tendons are exposed at the pes anserinus and divided at their musculotendinous junctions. Two large transverse holes are drilled though the patella and an oblique hole in the tibial tubercle. The autografts are placed though the holes in opposite directions and sutured together. Wire is then passed through the same holes under tension to protect the repair [38].

8.3.6 Complications

Delayed surgical repair of an acute patellar tendon rupture is associated with an adverse functional outcome [5, 9]. However, there are cases of neglected ruptures (up to 2 months in some cases) in the literature, which have been treated operatively and returned to previous levels of function [37].

8.4 Tibial Tubercle Avulsion Fractures

8.4.1 Epidemiology

Avulsion fractures of the tibial tubercle are rare accounting for less than 1 % of all physeal injuries [39]. It is usually found in adolescent boys who are nearing skeletal maturity [13]. The non-dominant leg is nearly always affected.

8.4.2 Aetiology

A reflex quadriceps contraction during a jump or fall is typically what results in this injury. Preceding history of Osgood Schlatter disease is a pre-disposing factor [40]. Injury is associated with sporting activities which involve jumping such as basketball or high jump [5].

8.4.3 Management

If displacement is less than 5 mm and the extensor mechanism intact, treatment is non-surgical [1]. The limb is cast immobilised in extension for 6 weeks and allowed to partially weight-bear.

Displaced fractures and those which have disrupted the articular surface require anatomical reduction and internal fixation [40, 41].

8.4.4 Complications

Prominence of the tibial tubercle and recurvatum following early physeal closure are rare complications.

These injuries when treated appropriately have excellent outcomes, with the majority able to return to previous levels of activity [40–42].

8.5 Extensor Mechanism Injuries Following Total Knee Arthroplasty

Injuries to the extensor mechanism following total knee arthroplasty (TKA) are associated with poor functional outcomes. Patients may experience recurrent falls, altered gait patterns and early prosthetic failure [43].

8.5.1 Quadriceps and Patellar Tendon Rupture

Patellar tendon rupture following TKA is uncommon with a reported incidence ranging from 0.7 to 2.5 % [44]. Quadriceps tendon rupture is even less frequent.

Over-resection of the patella with subsequent compromise at its proximal insertion pre-disposes to quadriceps tendon rupture. Previous tendon degeneration and lateral release (owing to damage to the superolateral genicular artery) increase the likelihood of this injury [45].

Risk factors for patellar tendon rupture include a pre-operative stiff knee, use of small incisions, a revision procedure, previous extensor mechanism repairs and systemic disease such as rheumatoid arthritis and immunosuppression [43].

Patellar tendon rupture may occur intraoperatively as a result of overzealous dissection or failure to protect the tendon during the tibial cut [45].

Hypovascularity is considered a major cause of late presentation, often 1–2 years after primary TKA. Devascularisation occurs as a result of a medial parapatellar approach (sacrifices 3 out of 4 of the genicular vessels) and excision of the fat pad [46].

Other causes include trauma, manipulation under anaesthetic and implant-related factors. If the tibial insert is too thick, it may cause shearing of the tendon at its anterior edge during deep flexion [44].

Surgery is always indicated unless the patient is medically unfit. Primary repairs of patellar tendon rupture following TKA alone are functionally poor [47]. Alternative techniques include semitendinosus autografts, a medial gastrocnemius muscle transposition flap, achilles tendon allografts and composite grafts [43, 44].

Emerson et al. described the use of an entire extensor mechanism allograft comprising quadriceps tendon, patella, patellar tendon and tibial tubercle [48]. The allograft tibial bone block is first secured to the host tibia with screws or cerclage wires. After ensuring satisfactory position of patella the host quadriceps is sutured to the allograft proximally. The repair should be tensioned in full extension and patella not resurfaced to avoid failure [43, 48–50]. The limb is immobilised in full extension for 6–8 weeks [44]. Extensor mechanism allograft is an attractive option as it does not rely on an intact patella and case series have shown good results following this repair with no extensor lag and full active extension in the majority of patients, although one isolated case series reported a 100 % failure rate [43, 50–52].

8.5.2 Periprosthetic Patellar Fracture

Periprosthetic patellar fracture in TKA is rare although rates vary from 0.68 % to 21 % [53]. The incidence is higher in resurfaced patellae.

The relatively high joint reaction forces at the PFJ are a key factor in the majority of patellofemoral complications following TKA [54]. High levels of activity, male gender, obesity, patellar thickness, component malalignment and poor implant design (metal-backed uncemented patellar component or those with a large central peg) are known predisposing factors [55, 56]. Avascular necrosis of the patella as a consequence of devascularisation following TKA surgery increases probability of fracture [57].

The AO Trauma Universal Classification System (UCS) for periprosthetic fractures categorises patellar fractures in the context of TKA into two main types [58].

Type A involves fractures at either the proximal (A1) or distal (A2) pole of the patella without loosening of the patellar component itself. In the presence of extensor mechanism, disruption surgical repair of the rupture is advocated with or without partial patellectomy.

Type B1 fractures comprise a non-displaced transverse fracture, well-fixed component and intact extensor mechanism which may be treated non-operatively. B2 and B3 fractures suggest loosening of the patellar component; however, the latter is complicated by substantial bone loss. In these circumstances the loose component should be removed to facilitate fracture fixation and extensor mechanism repair. Patellar resection arthroplasty must be considered in cases of significant bone loss.

8.5.3 Patellar Instability/Subluxation

Patellar instability and maltracking is the commonest complication after TKA with an incidence of 29 % [54].

The lateral force vector produced by the angle of pull of the quadriceps (Quadriceps 'Q' Angle) on the patella and tibial tubercle in extension pre-disposes to lateral dislocation. Patellar instability (PI) following TKA is reliant on maintenance of the normal Q angle. The major causes for PI include pre-operative valgus alignment of the knee, component malrotation, medialisation of either components and weak VMO or strong vastus lateralis muscle [54, 59].

Internal rotation of the femoral component medialises the trochlear, which increases the Q angle and likewise, internal rotation of the tibial component lateralises the tibial tubercle predisposing to subluxation [60].

Trial reduction is essential for assessment of patellar tracking and instability. A lateral release is commonly performed if instability is found intra-operatively, however, if there was no pre-operative instability, it is unlikely to be improved by a lateral release alone. Instead, external rotation of the tibial component or mediatisation of the tibial tubercle is recommended [59].

8.6 Conclusions

The extensor mechanism of the knee is essential for everyday functioning such as ambulation, standing from a seated position and walking up and down stairs. Injury to the extensor mechanism can be potentially devastating to everyday life. Disorders of the knee extensor apparatus may arise at any level. This chapter has discussed rupture of the quadriceps and patellar tendon, and tibial tubercle avulsion fractures. Disruption of the extensor mechanism in the context of total knee arthroplasty invariably will lead to unfavourable functional outcomes and subsequent poor prognoses, following what is usually a hugely successful procedure. Current treatment methods have been described, including the use of extensor mechanism allografts.

References

1. Sivananthan S, Sherry E, Warnke P, Miller MD (2012) Mercer's textbook of orthopaedics and trauma, 10th edn. Edward Arnold, London, pp 368–497
2. Archdeacon MT, Sanders RW (2009) Patella fractures and extensor mechanism injuries. Skeletal trauma basic science, management, and reconstruction, 4th edn. Saunders Elsevier Inc, Philadelphia, pp 2013–2015
3. Ilan DI, Tejwani N, Keschner M, Leibman M (2003) Quadriceps tendon rupture. J Am Acad Orthop Surg 11:192–200
4. Scuderi GR, Aglietti P, Menchetti PPM (1995) Biomechanics of the patellofemoral joint. The patella: Springer-Verlag, New York Inc, pp 25–29
5. Solomon L, Warwick DJ, Nayagam S (2001) Apley's system of orthopaedics and fractures, 8th edn. Arnold, London, pp 714–717
6. Trobisch PD, Bauman M, Weise K, Stuby F, Hak DJ (2010) Histologic analysis of ruptured quadriceps tendons. Knee Surg Sports Traumatol Arthrosc 18:85–88
7. Miller MD (2008) Review of orthopaedics, 5th edn. Saunders Elsevier Inc, Philadelphia, pp 618–621
8. Shah MK (2002) Simultaneous bilateral rupture of quadriceps tendons: analysis of risk factors and associations. South Med J 95:860–866
9. Egol AE, Koval KJ, Zuckerman JD (2010) Handbook of fractures, 4th edn. Lippincott Williams and Wilkins, Philadelphia, pp 439–452
10. Waligora AC, Johanson NA, Hirsch BE (2009) Clinical anatomy of the quadriceps femoris and extensor apparatus of the knee. Clin Orthop Relat Res 467:297–306
11. LaRocco BG, Zlupko G, Sierzenski P (2008) Ultrasound diagnosis of quadriceps tendon rupture. J Emerg Med 35:293–295
12. Puranik GS, Faraj A (2006) Outcome of quadriceps tendon repair. Acta Orthop Belgica 72:176–178
13. McRae R (2006) Pocketbook of orthopaedics and fractures, 2nd edn. Churchill Livingstone Elsevier, Philadelphia, pp 454–455
14. Kaneko K, DeMouy EH, Brunet ME, Benzian J (1994) Radiographic diagnosis of quadriceps tendon rupture: analysis of diagnostic failure. J Emerg Med 12:225–229
15. Seyahi A, Atalar AC, Koyuncu LO, Cinar BM, Demirhan M (2006) Blumensaat line and patellar height. Acta Orthop Traumatol Turcica 40:240–247
16. Rogers BA, Thornton-Bott P, Cannon SR, Briggs TW (2006) Interobserver variation in the measurement of patellar height after total knee arthroplasty. J Bone Joint Surg Br 88:484–488
17. Heyde CE, Mahlfeld K, Stahel PF, Kayser R (2005) Ultrasonography as a reliable diagnostic tool in old quadriceps tendon ruptures: a prospective multicentre study. Knee Surg Sports Traumatol Arthrosc 13:564–568
18. Siwek CW, Rao JP (1981) Ruptures of the extensor mechanism of the knee joint. J Bone Joint Surg Am 63:932–937
19. Wenzl ME, Kirchner R, Seide K, Strametz S, Jurgens C (2004) Quadriceps tendon ruptures-is there a complete functional restitution? Injury 35:922–926
20. Hak DJ, Sanchez A, Trobisch P (2010) Quadriceps tendon injuries. Orthopedics 33:40–46
21. Ramseier LE, Werner CM, Heinzelmann M (2006) Quadriceps and patellar tendon rupture. Injury 37:516–519
22. O'Shea K, Kenny P, Donovan J, Condon F, McElwain JP (2002) Outcomes following quadriceps tendon ruptures. Injury 33:257–260
23. Bartalena T, Rinaldi MF, De Luca C, Rimondi E (2010) Patellar tendon rupture: radiologic and ultrasonographic findings. West J Emerg Med 11:90–91
24. Sivananthan S, Sherry E, Warnke P, Miller MD (2012) Mercer's textbook of orthopaedics and trauma, 10th edn. Edward Arnold, London, pp 791–792
25. Bulstrode C, Buckwalter J, Carr A et al (2002) Oxford textbook of orthopaedics and trauma. vol 3, 1st edn. Oxford University Press Inc, New York, pp 1787–1788
26. Pang J, Shen S, Pan WR, Jones IR, Rozen WM, Taylor GI (2009) The arterial supply of the patellar tendon: anatomical study with clinical implications for knee surgery. Clin Anat 22:371–376
27. Canale ST (2003) Campbell's operative orthopaedics, vol 3, 10th edn. Mosby Inc, Philadelphia, pp. 2469–2470

28. Matava MJ (1996) Patellar tendon ruptures. J Am Acad Orthop Surg 4:287–296
29. Rasmussen OS (2000) Sonography of tendons. Scand J Med Science Sports 10:360–364
30. Miller MD, DeBerardino TM, Owens BD (2011) Repair of acute and chronic patellar tendon ruptures operative techniques in sports medicine surgery. Lippincott Williams and Wilkins, Philadelphia, pp 396–398
31. Karlsson J, Lundin O, Lossing IW, Peterson L (1991) Partial rupture of the patellar ligament. results after operative treatment. Am J Sports Med 19:403–408
32. Cooper ME, Selesnick FH (2000) Partial rupture of the distal insertion of the patellar tendon. a report of two cases in professional athletes. Am J Sports Med 28:402–406
33. Karlsson J, Kalebo P, Goksor LA, Thomee R, Sward L (1992) Partial rupture of the patellar ligament. Am J Sports Med 20:390–395
34. Lieberman JR (2009) AAOS comprehensive orthopaedic review american academy of orthopaedic surgeons. Rosemont, Illinois, pp 1101–1109
35. Marder RA, Timmerman LA (1999) Primary repair of patellar tendon rupture without augmentation. Am J Sports Med 27:304–307
36. Beavis RC, Barber FA (2009) Surgical management of acute patellar tendon rupture. Tech Knee Surg 8:194–200
37. Shepard GJ, Christodoulou L, Hegab AI (1999) Neglected rupture of the patellar tendon. Arch Orthop Trauma Surg 119:241–242
38. Ecker ML, Lotke PA, Glazer RM (1979) Late reconstruction of the patellar tendon. J Bone Joint Surg Am 61:884–886
39. Flynn JM (2011) Orthopaedic knowledge update, vol 10. AAOS, USA, pp 756–785
40. Zrig M, Annabi H, Ammari T, Trabelsi M, Mbarek M, Ben Hassine H (2008) Acute tibial tubercle avulsion fractures in the sporting adolescent. Arch Orthop Trauma Surg 128:1437–1442
41. Chow SP, Lam JJ, Leong JC (1990) Fracture of the tibial tubercle in the adolescent. J Bone Joint Surg Br 72:231–234
42. McKoy BE, Stanitski CL (2003) Acute tibial tubercle avulsion fractures. Orthop Clin North Am 34:397–403
43. Bernstein M, Bergeron SG, Antoniou J (eds) (2009) Extensor mechanism deficiency in total knee arthroplasty. Seminar Arthroplasty Elsevier, Philadelphia
44. Lonner JH, John T (eds) (2011) Extensor mechanism allografting. Seminar Arthroplasty Elsevier, Philadelphia
45. Brooks P, Higuera CA, Barsoum WK (eds) (2009) Prevention of intraoperative extensor mechanism injury in total knee arthroplasty. Seminars arthroplasty. Elsevier, Philadelphia
46. Lynch AF, Rorabeck CH, Bourne RB (1987) Extensor mechanism complications following total knee arthroplasty. J Arthroplasty 2:135–140
47. Kulkarni S, Sawant M, Ireland J (1999) Allograft reconstruction of the extensor mechanism for progressive extensor lag after total knee arthroplasty and previous patellectomy: a 3-year follow-up. J Arthroplasty 14:892–894
48. Emerson RH Jr, Head WC, Malinin TI (1990) Reconstruction of patellar tendon rupture after total knee arthroplasty with an extensor mechanism allograft. Clin Orthop Relat Res 260:154–161
49. Burnett RS, Berger RA, Paprosky WG, Della Valle CJ, Jacobs JJ, Rosenberg AG (2004) Extensor mechanism allograft reconstruction after total knee arthroplasty. A comparison of two techniques. J Bone Joint Surg Am 86:2694–2699
50. Nazarian DG, Booth RE Jr (1999) Extensor mechanism allografts in total knee arthroplasty. Clin Orthop Relat Res 367:123–129
51. Emerson RH Jr, Head WC, Malinin TI (1994) Extensor mechanism reconstruction with an allograft after total knee arthroplasty. Clin Orthop Relat Res 303:79–85
52. Leopold SS, Greidanus N, Paprosky WG, Berger RA, Rosenberg AG (1999) High rate of failure of allograft reconstruction of the extensor mechanism after total knee arthroplasty. J Bone Joint Surg Am 81:1574–1579
53. Ortiguera CJ, Berry DJ (2002) Patellar fracture after total knee arthroplasty. J Bone Joint Surg Am 84:532–540
54. Rhee S, Haddad F (2008) Patello-femoral joint in total knee replacement. Curr Orthop 22:132–138
55. Austin MS, de Jesus D (2006) Patella fracture after total knee arthroplasty. Semin Arthroplasty 17:6–8
56. Healy WL, Wasilewski SA, Takei R, Oberlander M (1995) Patellofemoral complications following total knee arthroplasty. correlation with implant design and patient risk factors. J Arthroplasty 10:197–201
57. Ritter MA, Herbst SA, Keating EM, Faris PM, Meding JB (1996) Patellofemoral complications following total knee arthroplasty. effect of a lateral release and sacrifice of the superior lateral geniculate artery. J Arthroplasty 11:368–372
58. Haddad FS, Duncan C (2013) Peri-prosthetic Fractures. In: Ruedi T (ed) Manual of internal fixation: techniques recommended by the AO group. (In Press)
59. Briard JL, Hungerford DS (1989) Patellofemoral instability in total knee arthroplasty. J Arthroplasty 4:S87–S97
60. Hungerford DS. Technical factors contributing to patellar instability in TKA. Semins Arthroplasty. 21:129–133

9 Meniscus Tears

Julián Fernández-González, Santiago J. Ponce and Ruben Fole

9.1 Introduction

Meniscal injuries are probably the most common injuries of the knee. It is well known for the important role of the meniscus in the stability and function of the knee, especially since Fairbanks description. Total and partial meniscectomy often lead to degenerative cartilage injury, flattening of the articular surfaces, subchondral bone sclerosis, and marginal osteophyte formation. In several years this changes manifest clinically [1, 2].

Meniscal tears could happen at any age, but in our experience we must distinguish meniscal tears according to the age of the patient: young people (<40 years), middle-age (40–65 years), and people over 65 years. The type of tear and its treatment will be related to the patient's age, which is also associated with physical activity and type of job.

Morphology of the tear is also related to patient age, being longitudinal injuries the most frequent type of tears found in young patients and degenerative tears in people over 40 years. Degenerative tears over 40 years of age are produced with banal daily movements of the knee.

J. Fernández-González (✉) · S. J. Ponce · R. Fole
Department of Orthopaedic Surgery,
Hospital Universitario La Princesa, Diego de León 62, 28006, Madrid, Spain
e-mail: julfergon@hotmail.com

9.2 Anatomy and Biomechanics

The menisci are fibro-cartilaginous structures, with a semilunar morphology in the horizontal plane and wedge in the frontal plane.

The menisci occupy 60 % of the contact area between the articular surfaces and transmit more than 50 % of the compressive forces generated in the joint. After meniscectomy, the tibiofemoral contact surface covered by meniscus decreases by 50 %, and the contact forces are increased by 2 to 3 times [2, 3].

It can be defined in three anatomical areas, each one with clinical differences: anterior root, body, and posterior root. The posterior root is the most common site of meniscal tears and the more symptomatic. Anterior root lesions are rare and usually produce fewer symptoms; however complete injuries or removal can produce an unstable meniscus. This occurs especially in the lateral meniscus and produces pain and functional impairment.

The menisci are attached to the joint capsule in most of its extension, and on the medial side they are attached to the deep layer of the medial collateral ligament. The lateral meniscus in its posterolateral region is not adhered to the joint capsule, to facilitate passage of the popliteal tendon.

Morphology of the lateral meniscus is more variable than the medial meniscus, the former can have a discoid shape, and sometimes it has an incomplete union in the posterior root area, forming the Wrisberg's discoid meniscus.

E. C. Rodríguez-Merchán (ed.), *Traumatic Injuries of the Knee*,
DOI: 10.1007/978-88-470-5298-7_9, © Springer-Verlag Italia 2013

Its composition and arrangement of type I collagen fibers are essential for understanding the behavior and action. In the periphery there is predomination of longitudinal fibers, which are disposed from the posterior to the anterior root, primarily resisting compression forces. In the center, fibers are arranged in a radial distribution, which resist tension forces.

Another important aspect is meniscal vascularization, remembering that the outermost third of them is irrigated by terminal branches of the medial and lateral geniculate arteries. The two inner thirds are avascular, which explains the difficulty of primary healing or secondary repair [4].

Following this vascularization pattern, meniscal tears can be classified into inner third tears (avascular white-white area), medial third tears (white-red area, the vessels reach the external area of this region, approximately 4 mm from its peripheral insertion), and peripheral or external third tears (vascularized or red-red area) [2, 3]. Vessel arrangement plays an important role in the prognosis and treatment of meniscal injuries.

The menisci are innervated, emphasizing proprioceptive innervation, which reports the position of the knee at all times and helps on defense maneuvering during motion.

9.3 Clinical Findings

Clinical findings in meniscal lesions depend upon patient's age. In most cases there is a traumatic etiology, and in many other cases a rotational mechanism. It is common tibio-femoral joint-line tenderness and pain and its extension to the posterior region.

In young patients symptoms are pain and functional impairment, sometimes associated with a lack of full extension. It is frequent that in 12–24 h an articular effusion takes place and depending on its volume can cause a knee with an attitude in flexion that can be confused with a true locking. This attitude in flexion is solved after an arthrocentesis, which usually yields inflammatory fluid, and is accompanied by significant pain relief. Whenever there is a suspected meniscal injury the physician must perform a thorough physical examination to rule out associated chondral and ligamentous injuries.

Rupture of the anterior cruciate ligament (ACL) is associated with meniscal tears in 40–60 % of the patients, being the lateral meniscus the most frequent injured [5]. Most of these injuries can be managed with conservative treatment, being incomplete or small (< 1 cm) injuries. These injuries may be repaired when they are unstable or larger than 1 cm which occur in the peripheral third of the meniscus [2, 3].

Patients between 40 and 60-years old, injuries are degenerative, caused by trauma or knee movements typically done in daily life. The main complain is pain and variable functional impairment in the first 4–6 weeks. Beyond this period of time, pain may persist, but most of the patients improve of the previous state of functional disability. The decision to address surgical treatment is dependent upon each patient, depending on their symptoms and disability after this period of time.

In patients over 65 years, it is common that meniscal injuries are accompanied with chondral lesions, the latter being the ones that primarily cause symptoms and functional impairment at medium term. The clinical findings are similar to the previous group, knee pain for 4–6 weeks, being very common to experience great improvement or fully resolution of symptoms in 3–4 months.

In most meniscal lesions is important to rest for 1 week and maintain partial weight bearing, except for injuries that produce knee locking since the beginning. From the first day patients should perform isometric exercises which prevent the development of muscle atrophy (quadriceps muscle), which is sometimes more responsible for functional impairment than the primary meniscal injury.

9.4 Classification

Meniscal injuries can be classified either by their morphology, location, or by its size, being the size an important factor in the stability of the injury.

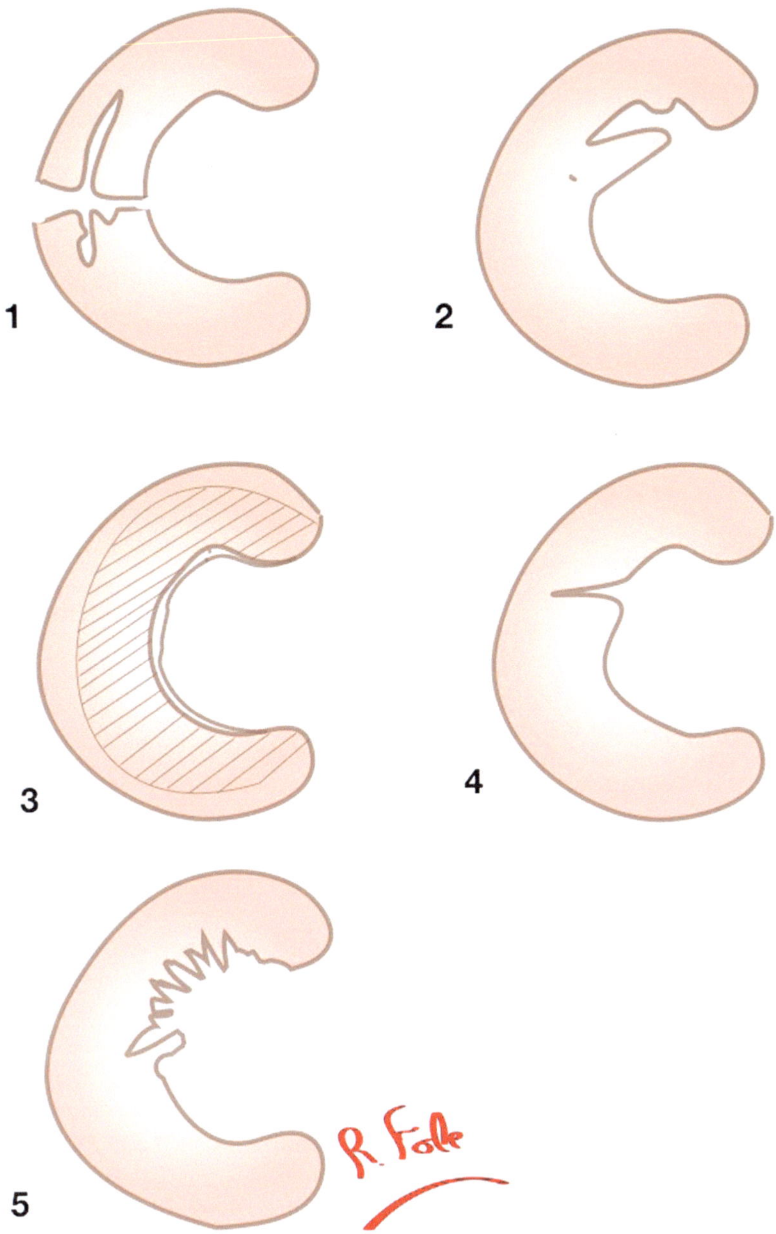

Fig. 9.1 Patterns of meniscal tears: bucket-handle (**1**), flap (**2**), horizontal (**3**), radial (**4**) and degenerative (**5**)

Figure 9.1 shows the different types of tears. Longitudinal lesions occur mainly in the second and third decades of life. Degenerative injuries which are predominantly horizontal occur beyond the fourth decade, being favored by the degenerative process of the meniscus.

Regarding localization, as we have mentioned previously, we can differentiate injuries that occur in the peripheral zone of the meniscus which is well irrigated, and those in the avascular medial area [4].

The size or extent of the injury will be responsible for the degree of stability, considering stable injuries the ones that are less than 1 cm, more than 1 cm potentially unstable and more than 2–3 cm clearly unstable [2, 3].

9.5 Physical Examination

There are multiple tests described in the literature to examine the menisci. The most commonly performed are: forced flexion plus varus and internal rotation to test medial meniscus injuries, and compression, valgus and external rotation to test lateral meniscus lesions. This test is similar to the one described by Mc Murray, which is positive for posterior root injuries when it is accompanied by hearing a click that represents the movement of the torn meniscal fragment by the femoral condyle.

Physician should always test the coexistence of associated patellofemoral pathology or collateral ligaments injuries, predominantly the medial collateral ligament and ACL.

9.6 Imaging

Once there is clinically suspicion of meniscal injury, X-rays should be performed including a posteroanterior and lateral view, the former view should be weight bearing. Full-length standing hip-knee-ankle weight-bearing radiographs may rule out lower limb malalignment in the frontal plane, either varus or valgus, which favors the existence of chondral lesions and also helps in decision making toward treatment.

MRI (Magnetic Resonance Imaging) confirms the existence of a meniscal injury, and rules out the existence of associated injuries. Thus, MRI in young people confirms meniscal injury and helps to rule out traumatic chondral or osteochondral lesions. In middle-aged people and especially females, it helps to rule out osteonecrosis which often presents with a clinical pattern similar to meniscal tears.

After traumatic injuries, MRI helps to rule out ligament injuries, especially injuries of the medial collateral ligament and anterior cruciate ligament. These ligaments lesions are much more common than injuries to the posterolateral corner structures of the knee. MRI can also exclude as a source of pain, stress fractures of the medial tibial plateau, sometimes mistaken for medial meniscus injuries (Fig. 9.2a and b).

MRI should always be performed after a true suspicion of meniscal injury, since there are a lot of clinical studies about asymptomatic patients with meniscal tears. It helps to define the type and size of the injury, especially in cases of instability or bucket handle cases to consider the possibility of meniscal repair (Fig. 9.3a, b and c).

9.7 Treatment

Most meniscal lesions are treated arthroscopically. However, meniscal repair can be arthroscopically assisted (inside-out, outside-in) in different ways (Figs. 9.4a and b, 9.5, 9.6a, b, c, and d) and all-arthroscopic.

The treatment of injuries will depend on the type, location, and size of the tear. Certainly, today is widely believed that whenever possible, the meniscal lesion should be repaired instead of a meniscectomy.

As mentioned previously, in most lesions a partial meniscectomy is performed, as in degenerative lesions or in non-degenerative lesions which do not reach the peripheral well irrigated outer third.

Repair of the meniscal lesion should be performed in non-degenerative tears that compromise the vascularized area: suturing can be done with three different techniques: "outside-in", "inside-out", or "all-inside," being the latter the most frequent technique which is done with arthroscopy with different repair systems. In our experience, it is possible to combine different surgical techniques: meniscal fixator devices or sutured-based devices for posterior root and meniscal body tears, and inside-out or outside-in suture repair techniques for anterior root injuries.

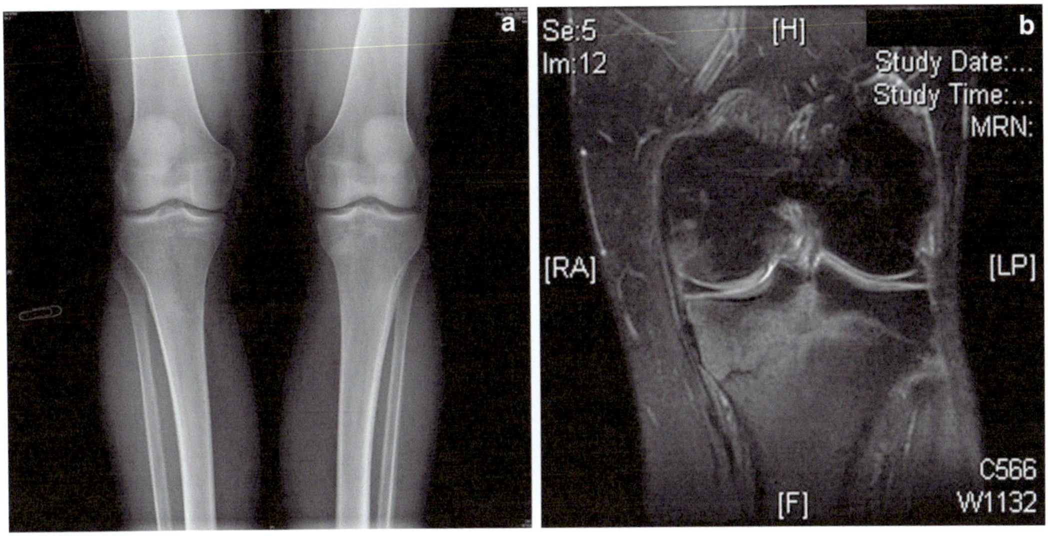

Fig. 9.2 Male patient with medial pain in his left knee. He suddenly suffered acute onset of pain in his left knee after a race. In this case medial pain was localized to the medial tibial metaphysis and also to the medial joint line. (**a**) At first glance, posteroanterior weight bearing X–rays do not show any bone lesion. (**b**) MRI done following 4 weeks of the incident. The patient continued with persistent knee pain. Coronal image shows a clear fracture line at the medial tibial metaphysis. These stress fractures of the medial tibial plateau, sometimes are mistaken for medial meniscus injuries

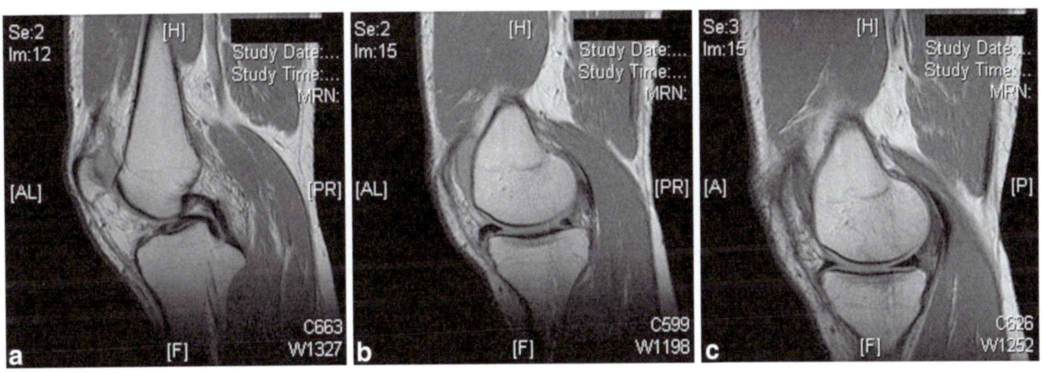

Fig. 9.3 MRI imaging of a patient who suffered a knee injury with an ACL rupture and a bucket–handle tear of the medial meniscus. In this case MRI provides important information regarding the type of meniscal tear and the potential for repair it. (**a**) Sagital view that shows the medial fragment of the medial meniscus at the intercondylar area. (**b**) Another sagittal MRI view that shows the small posterior root remaining of the medial meniscus in that longitudinal rupture. (**c**) MRI sagital imaging done after ACL reconstruction and meniscal medial repair. It shows integrity and shape recovery of the posterior root of the medial meniscus

Other clear indications of meniscal repair are: when coexistence of other ligament injuries, primarily ACL; associated traumatic joint injuries while reconstructing ligaments; reducible meniscal tears with a good quality fragment and proper meniscal irrigation of the fragment, which can be determined by the existence of bleeding while shaving, and simple pattern tears (longitudinal or radial) in the inner area that extend to the peripheral well-irrigated area [2, 3].

Borderline indications are complex tears, multiple plane tears that affect both the central and peripheral areas of the meniscus [2].

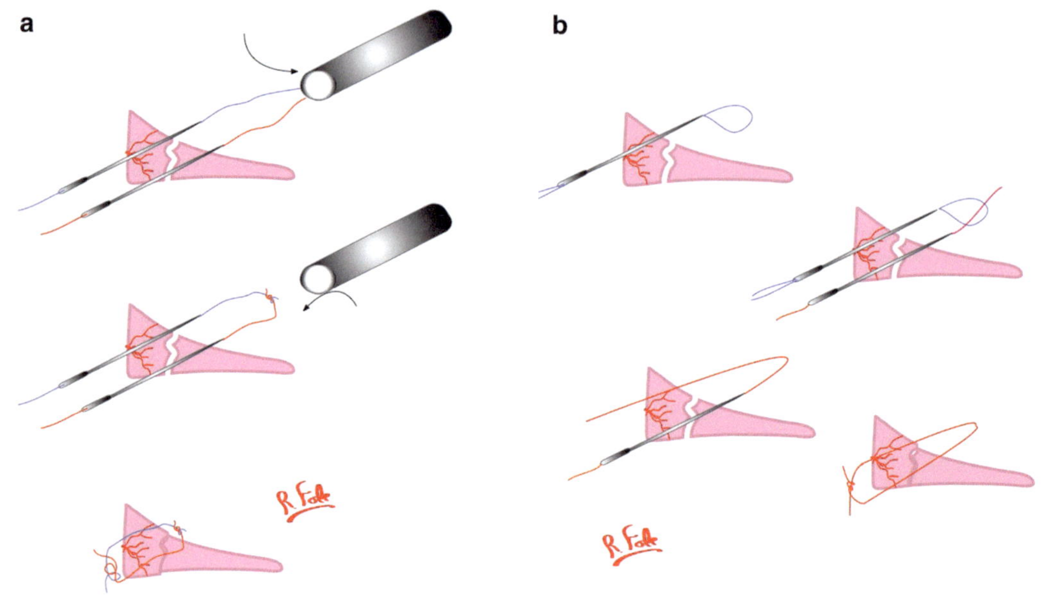

Fig. 9.4 Two different ways (**a**, **b**) to perform an outside-in suture technique

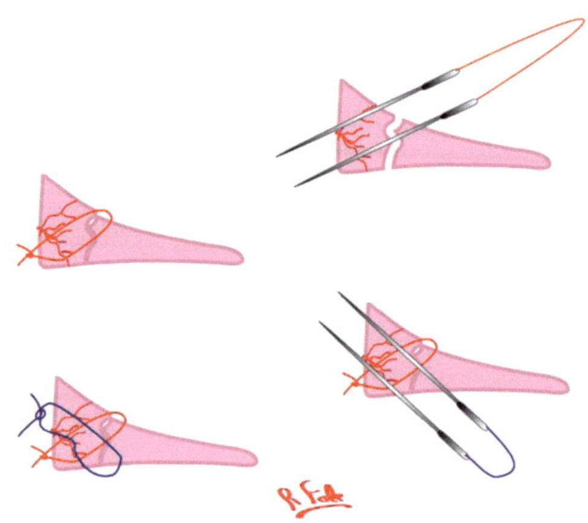

Fig. 9.5 Inside–out suture technique: double–stacked vertical suture used for repair of longitudinal meniscal tears

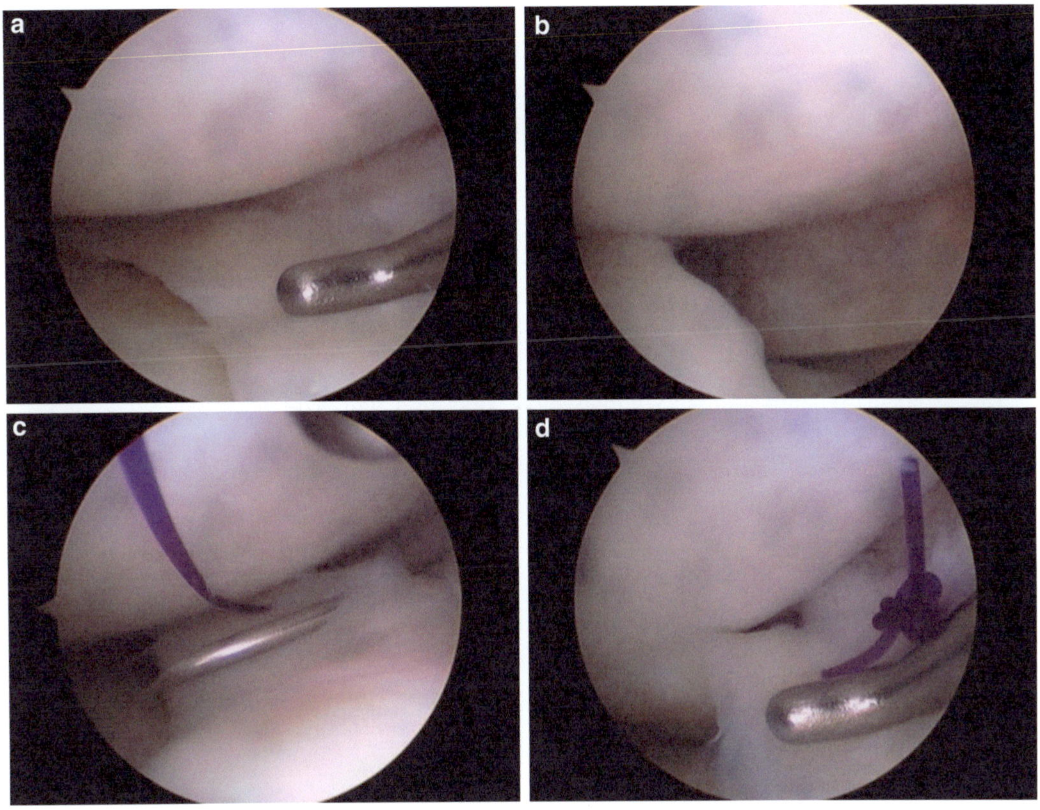

Fig. 9.6 Arthroscopic views of a medial meniscus repair with sutures ("out–inside" technique). (**a**) Arthroscopic view that shows the longitudinal peripheral tear of the medial meniscus. (**b**) Note the peripheral tear and its clear instability. (**c**) After rasping of the vascularized parameniscal synovium, action that can encourage the meniscal repair, one step of the suture surgical technique is shown. (**d**) Final arthroscopic view showing two of the four "outside–in" sutures done in this meniscal repair

Contraindications: joint space narrowing and/or existence of Fairbanks signs; increased varus above normal (>3° varus) for medial lesions and valgus (>7°) for lesions of the lateral meniscus; diffuse lesions grade 3 and 4 of the ICRS (International Cartilage Repair Society) while performing arthroscopy (Table 9.1) [6]. Regarding to the type of meniscal tear: injuries in the avascular zone of the meniscus; complex degenerative injuries or tears with bad quality meniscal tissue; radial tears that do not reach the well-irrigated zone or small (<1 cm) stable longitudinal tears [2, 3].

Another important aspect in the decision making process is the patient's compromise with a long rehabilitation program, and to renounce significant physical activity or sports for at least 4–6 months.

There are several surgical techniques described to treat symptomatic isolated tears of the posterior root of the medial meniscus in young patients, some of them of great difficulty [7].

9.8 Clinical Outcome of Meniscal Repair

9.8.1 Inside-Out Repair Technique

Arthroscopically assisted inside-out repair techniques have been termed the gold standard of meniscal repair [2].

Table 9.1 ICRS (International Cartilage Repair Society) classification system [6]

Grade	
Grade 0	Macroscopically normal cartilage
Grade Ia	Cartilage with an intact surface with fibrillation and/or slight softening
Grade Ib	Grade Ia with additional superficial lacerations and fissures
Grade II	Defects that extend deeper but involve less than 50 % of the cartilage thickness
Grade III	Defects that extend more than 50 % of the cartilage thickness, but not through the subchondral bone plate
Grade IV	Cartilage lesions that extend into the subchondral bone

This technique requires accessory portals for a safe suture retrieval, either a posteromedial or a posterolateral ones. These small (3 cm) approaches can protect the neurovascular structures of the popliteal fossa, while performing the suture knot.

A double-stacked vertical suture is recommended for the repair of longitudinal meniscal tears, on the upper edge of the tear and on the bottom edge. It is recommended to space the sutures at least 3–5 mm. The superior suture reduces the meniscus to its bed and the inferior sutures close the inferior gap of the tear [2] (Fig. 9.5).

In radial tears, transverse sutures are recommended, placing first the most inner sutures. Generally 2–3 upper sutures and two lower sutures are enough [2].

In flap tears, horizontal tension sutures are placed to reduce the radial component and the longitudinal part is sutured with use of the double-stacked suture technique [2].

Several studies have shown the clinical results of this suture technique. Evidence shows good results of meniscal repair with this technique while performing an ACL reconstruction. The authors report satisfactory clinical results in injuries that occur in the vascularized area (94 %), but these positive healing results decrease to 54 % in complete tears of the central area [8].

One prospective study reported a reoperation rate of 20 % because of tibiofemoral symptoms of the repaired tears which extended into the middle third of the meniscus or that had a rim width of 4 mm or more. In this study the effect of six factors on healing rates of meniscal repair were evaluated. One conclusion was that the lateral meniscus repair is more likely to heal than the medial meniscus [9].

There is another prospective study to assess the age of the patients at the time of making a decision to perform a meniscal suture. In this paper the patients who were treated were >40 years old with tears that extended to the avascular area. In 87 % of the patients, it was unnecessary to perform a second surgery. The outcome was not influenced by which compartment was affected, the chronicity of the injury, concomitant ACL reconstruction, or the status of the articular cartilage [10].

9.8.2 All-Arthroscopic Repair Technique

This technique has been designed to carry out these repairs there are systems that integrate anchors with sutures and others which are just anchors without suture material. This is performed arthroscopically.

The majority of these arthroscopic repairs allow the surgeon to give compression across the tear site, while avoid performing additional portals in order to prevent neurovascular injury [3].

Systems incorporating sutures have shown good biomechanically results approaching those of vertical sutures placed inside-out, and better outcomes than when using implants without sutures [3] (Fig. 9.7a, b and c).

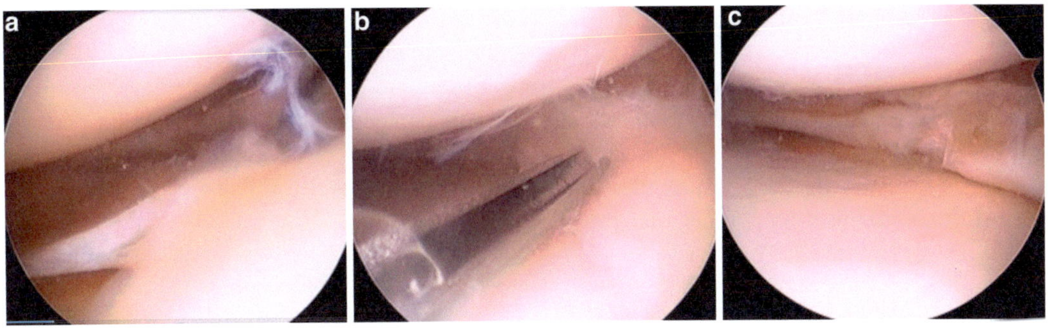

Fig. 9.7 Arthroscopic views of a medial meniscus repair with a suture-based device. (**a**) In this case, the arthroscopic view show a complex medial meniscus tear, with a radial and a longitudinal component. (**b**) This image shows one step of the technique consisting of the placement of a soft-tissue anchor in an extracapsular position through a needle delivery system at the anterior part of the longitudinal meniscus tear. (**c**) Final result of the meniscal repair, with two sutures-based devices in the posterior root of meniscus and one in the anterior part of the longitudinal tear. In this case, every suture-based device has "a top hat" that compresses the meniscal tear against the extracapsular anchor with a connecting suture. Now, our trend is to combine both procedures (outside–in or inside–out suture techniques with suture-based devices) in meniscal repairs

Laboratory tests have shown that sutures are highly resistant to failure, most of them composed of ultra high molecular weight polyethylene.

Clinical results with one of these repair systems that include integrated locking sutures and anchor devices, have encouraging results, with a failure rate of 9–13 % [11, 12]. The clinical results were good for both isolated meniscal repairs and those associated with an ACL reconstruction [11]. With other type of system, a first generation integrated locking suture and anchor device, the authors obtained good results in 90.7 % of cases in which a concomitant ACL reconstruction was done [13]. The modification of the implant material of the previous system did not improve the results which were good in 86.8 % of cases, but there were no chondral lesions noted during four second-look arthroscopies [14].

The proponents of the suture repair technique inside-out believe that the use of 2 or 3 meniscal fixator devices or suture-based devices provide inadequate fixation when compared with the inside-out repair technique [2]. Thus, the results with these sutures appear to worsen over time. In our experience, it is convenient to combine the two techniques, which shortens the operating time of the inside-out repair procedure.

Local complications have been reported specially with first generation of these implants, as chondral lesion, cyst formation, repetitive joint effusions, synovitis, and breakage with extra-articular migration. These complications have been significantly decreased with the development of suture-based meniscal repair devices. The complication most specific to the suture-based device is soft-tissue irritation from the extracapsular placement of the anchors [3, 15].

9.9 Postoperative Rehabilitation

Rehabilitation of a meniscal repair requires a guided physical therapy protocol. Immediate movement of the knee is permitted from 0 to 90° in the first 2 weeks. Range of motion of 120° by 3–4 weeks, and 135° by 5–6 weeks. Partial weight bearing during the first 4–6 weeks is recommended. Squatting or forced knee flexion is not allowed for 4–6 months. Not running, jumping, or pivoting until 6 months [3].

9.10 Meniscal Transplantation

Not all torn menisci are repairable, especially if considerable tissue damage or a complex tear has occurred. Meniscal transplantation has been developed to restore the load-bearing function of the meniscus, decrease symptoms, and provide chondroprotective effects [2, 16, 17].

Meniscal transplantation has been described more than two decades ago [18]. It is an evolving technique, with good short-term results in terms of pain reduction, but the different existing clinical studies have shown that transplanted meniscus deteriorate over time, tear or suffer decrease in size and volume [2]. Therefore it requires to be performed in reference centers with experience.

Meniscal transplantation can be performed either by allografts cultured "in vitro" immediately removed from the donor, fresh frozen or cryopreserved allografts [2]. The idea of viable allograft transplants is to maintain alive cells and their ability to synthesize their extracellular matrix molecules in the culture system. These grafts must be implanted within 14 days, meanwhile presence of transmissible diseases is ruled out according to the International Tissue Bank Standards and to plan carefully the surgical procedure [16].

Meniscal transplantation is indicated for patients under 50 years old who had previously had a meniscectomy. The requirements are: marked symptoms with daily activities, the lack of femorotibial space narrowing over 50 % on weight-bearing x-ray, absence of osteophytes that prevent a good settlement of the meniscus; besides there should not be diffuse chondral lesions. The only acceptable chondral injuries are the ones that can be addressed at the same time of meniscal transplantation, either by microfracture technique, mosaicplasty, or chondrocyte implantation. Normal axial alignment and a stable joint are required. The body mass index must be within the normal range [2].

The main contraindications would be grade IV chondral injuries, marked degenerative signs such as flattening of the condyles or osteophyte formation, frontal plane deviations above normal, ligamentous instability, inflammatory joint disease, and previous history of infection [2].

There are prospective studies of fresh-frozen irradiated meniscal allografts. In one of these studies with a mean follow-up of 44 months (22–111), almost 30 % failed early, and the rest of the patients have good pain relief with daily activities [19]. This study recommended not performing this procedure in patients with advanced arthritis and alterations in joint geometry with exposed bone surfaces.

Another prospective study with cryopreserved meniscal allografts there was 30 % of failure. Most patients experienced pain relieved in daily activities and 68 % had no tibiofemoral compartment pain, clinical sign presented in all patients preoperatively. 89 % stated that the condition of their knee had improved. There was displacement in the sagittal and coronal plane of the transplanted menisci measured by MRI [20].

Publications such as the ones of Verdonk et al. have shown promising results at long term, so at 10 years there is a satisfactory result in 70 % of the implanted grafts. From 100 fresh meniscal transplants, the failure rate of the medial side was 28 % and only 16 % on the lateral side, however the latter one had less mean time to failure. The survival of the medial meniscus was higher when a valgus osteotomy was associated (survival of 83 % at 10 years) [16].

So the main indication for meniscal transplantation would be a young people with pain in daily activities, as there are few alternatives. Short-term results are improvement in function and particularly in pain relief. However, it is unknown whether the transplanted meniscus has protective effects on the articular cartilage. Clinical results show that the beneficial effects diminish over time, and probably these patients may require further surgery in the future [2].

9.11 Treatments that Promote Repair of a Meniscal Tear

In meniscal injuries in the avascular area, healing could be promoted by different means, as with fibrin clot, which contributes with growth factors that promote chemotaxis and cell proliferation at the tear [3]. Another technique is perforations or trephination which reach the vascularized area, favoring the ingrowth of vessels, and cell migration to the tear site [3].

Both techniques can be combined by rasping of the vascularized parameniscal synovium. This procedure result in superior healing compared with that following the use of a fibrin clot [3]. Therefore, this action can encourage the good results in meniscal repair techniques.

Recently, PRP (platelet-rich plasma) has been used as an adjuvant for meniscal tears healing. It contains multiple growth factors, which may be more useful than using a specific isolated growth factor. The action of PRP seems to stimulate chemotaxis, cell proliferation, and angiogenesis. However, not all growth factors have shown the ability to promote repair of the meniscal lesion [3].

9.12 Conclusions

In summary, meniscal lesions should be approached with a repair technique as the first choice of treatment, especially in patients below 40–50 years, since performing a partial or total meniscectomy frequently leads to irreparable joint damage, including degeneration of the articular cartilage. It has been reported that, as early as 4.5 years after meniscectomy, degenerative changes can be seen on an X-ray, as flattening of the articular surfaces and subchondral bone sclerosis. Thus, when it is indicated, meniscal repair should be done meticulously. In some complex tears the surgical time could be similar to an ACL reconstruction surgery. Successful healing of meniscal repair may be achieved by biologic augmentation (the addition of a fibrin clot). Meniscal transplant should be performed in young patients with continuous pain in daily activities with no other surgical options.

References

1. Andersson-Molina H, Karlsson H, Rockborn P (2002) Arthroscopic partial and total meniscectomy: a long-term follow-up study with matched control. Arthroscopy 18:183–189
2. Noyes FR, Barber-Wenstin SD, Chen RC (2011) Repair of complex and avascular meniscal tears and meniscal Transplantation. In: Egol KA, Tornetta III P (eds) Instructional course lectures, vol 60. American Academy of Orthopaedic Surgeons, Rosemont Illinois, pp 415–437
3. Kessler MW, Sgaglione NA (2011) All-arthroscopic repair of avascular and biologically at-risk meniscal tears. In: Egol KA, Tornetta III P (eds) Instructional course lectures, vol 60. American Academy of Orthopaedic Surgeons, Rosemont Illinois, pp 439–452
4. Arnoczky SP, Warren RF (1982) Microvasculature of the human meniscus. Am J Sports Med 10:90–95
5. Noyes FR, Bassett RW, Grood ES, Butler DL (1980) Arthroscopy in acute traumatic hemarthrosis of the knee: incidence of anterior cruciate tears and other injuries. J Bone Joint Surg Am 62:687–695
6. Brittberg M, Winalski CS (2003) Evaluation of cartilage injuries and repair. J Bone Joint Surg Am 85(suppl 2):58–69
7. Harner CD, Mauro CS, Lesniak BP, Romanowski JR (2009) Biomechanical consequences of a tear of the posterior root of the medial meniscus. J Bone Joint Surg Am 91:257–270
8. Buseck MS, Noyes FR (1991) Arthroscopic evaluation of meniscal repairs after anterior cruciate ligament reconstruction and immediate motion. Am J Sports Med 19:489–494
9. Rubman MH, Noyes FR, Barber-Westin SD (1998) Arthroscopic repair of meniscal tears that extend into the avascular zone: a review of 198 single and complex tears. Am J Sports Med 26:87–95
10. Noyes FR, Barber-Westin SD (2000) Arthroscopic repair of meniscus tears extending into the avascular zone with or without anterior cruciate ligament reconstruction in patients 40 years of age and older. Arthroscopy 16:822–829
11. Kotsovolos ES, Hantes ME, Mastrokalos DS, Lorbach O, Paessler HH (2006) Results of all-inside meniscal repair with the FasT-Fix meniscal repair system. Arthroscopy 22:3–9
12. Barber FA, Schroeder FA, Oro FB, Beavis RC (2008) FasT-Fix meniscal repair: mid-term results. Arthroscopy 24:1342–1348
13. Quinby JS, Golish SR, Hart JA, Diduch DR (2006) All-inside meniscal repair using a new flexible, tensionable device. Am J Sports Med 34:1281–1286

14. Billante MJ, Diduch DR, Lunardini DJ, Treme GP, Miller MD, Hart JM (2008) Meniscal repair using an all-inside, rapidly absorbing, tensionable device. Arthroscopy 24:779–785
15. Sgaglione NA (2004) Complications of meniscus surgery. Sports Med Arthrosc 12:148–159
16. Verdonk PCM, Demurie A, Almqvist KF, Veys EM, Verbruggen G, Verdonk R (2006) Transplantation of viable meniscal allograft. J Bone Joint Surg Am 88:109–118
17. Szomor ZL, Martin TE, Bonar F, Murrell GA (2000) The protective effects of meniscal transplantation on cartilage: an experimental study in sheep. J Bone Joint Surg Am 82:80–88
18. Locht RC, Gross AE, Langer F (1984) Late osteochondral allograft resurfacing for tibial plateau fractures. J Bone Joint Surg Am 66:328–335
19. Noyes FR, Barber-Westin SD, Butler DL, Wilkins RM (1998) The role of allografts in repair and reconstruction of knee joint ligaments and menisci. Instructional Course Lectures, Rosemont Illinois 47:379–396
20. Noyes FR, Barber-Westin SD, Rankin M (2004) Meniscal transplantation in symptomatic patients less than fifty years old. J Bone Joint Surg Am 86:1392–1404

Anterior Cruciate Ligament (ACL) Injuries

10

Ana María Valverde-Villar, Primitivo Gómez-Cardero and E. Carlos Rodríguez-Merchán

10.1 Introduction

The first description of anterior cruciate ligament (ACL) is due to Galen [1] and Stark [2] in 1850, who described the first case of rupture of this ligament. In 1917, Hey-Groves [3], which can be considered father of ligamentoplasties, described the first intra-articular ACL reconstruction. ACL injury is the most common knee injury that requires a ligament reconstruction. It is the subject of many laboratory and clinical papers because there is controversy about its natural history and some aspects of its treatment like the graft selection, placement and fixation. In this chapter we will discuss current knowledge about the ACL-deficient knee and review the current studies in the literature about it.

10.2 Anatomy and Function

The ACL has an average length between 31 mm [4] and 38 mm [5] along its anterior border. It is composed of two bands: anteromedial band and posterolateral band [6]. The anteromedial band is tighter during positions of knee flexion (60–90°), while the posterolateral band is tighter during position of extension [7] but they function together throughout the arc of motion of the knee and serve as the primary restraint to anterior subluxation of the tibia on the femur, major secondary restraint to internal rotation and minor restraint to external rotation, varus and valgus forces [8]. It has been suggested that the ACL function as a sensory organ, not only providing propioceptive feedback but also initiating protective and stabilizing muscular reflexes [9].

For the surgeon, a correct understanding of the femoral and tibial insertions of the ACL is particularly important because a common cause for reconstructive failure is placement of the graft outside these insertions [10–12]. Anatomic placement of grafts has been identified as a key to improved surgical outcomes [13].

The tibial insertion lies between the medial and the lateral tubercles with oval shape and approximate length of 18 × 10 mm [6, 14, 15]. Debates occur indentifying anterior and posterior boundaries. The center of the tibial footprint is usually placed 7–15 mm anterior to the posterior cruciate ligament (PCL) [14, 16].

The femoral attachment in the posteromedial side of the lateral femoral condyle has similar footprint measurements than tibial [17]. Its posterior insertion is separated from the posterior articular cartilage of at most 4 mm and its anterior border lies directly anterior to a ringe on

A. M. Valverde-Villar (✉) · P. Gómez-Cardero · E. C. Rodríguez-Merchán
Department of Orthopaedic Surgery, "La Paz" University Hospital-Idipaz, Paseo de la Castellana, 261, 28046, Madrid, Spain
e-mail: anavavi@hotmail.com

P. Gómez-Cardero
e-mail: gcarderop@hotmail.com

E. C. Rodríguez-Merchán
e-mail: ecrmerchan@gmx.es

E. C. Rodríguez-Merchán (ed.), *Traumatic Injuries of the Knee*,
DOI: 10.1007/978-88-470-5298-7_10, © Springer-Verlag Italia 2013

the medial aspect of the condyle termed the resident's ringe. Visualizing the femoral insertion during an arthroscopic procedure can be difficult. Generally, the overhang of articular cartilage at the anterior border of the notch occults the posterior notch, and a notchplasty is necessary to gain a view of the ACL insertion.

Primary blood supply to the ligament comes from the middle genicular artery, with additional supply coming from the inferomedial and inferolateral genicular arteries [18].

10.3 Epidemiology

ACL injury is a common injury above in active people. The estimated United States incidence is 100,000–200,000 ACL tears per year [9]. Football players are the most affected population with skiers and gymnasts [19, 20]. Sports with sidestepping and crossover cutting maneuvers are the riskiest. Muscle weakness or fatigue, hyperlaxity as notch stenosis may contribute to increase the rates of injury [9]. The injury rates tend to be higher in women than for men [21–23] may be due to less strength in quadriceps, much laxity and more frequent notch stenosis.

In pediatric population these injuries have become relatively common with the increased extend of athletic activity over the last few decades [24]. The most frequent history of an ACL injury is a non-contact deceleration, jumping o cutting action, usually involving changing direction that produce rotational and lateral bending in valgus motion of the extended knee [25, 26]. A "pop" could be heard and/or felt. Swelling frequently appears and aspiration reveals hemarthrosis 3 or 4 h post-injury.

10.4 Diagnosis and Imaging

Physical examination frequently establishes a diagnosis of ACL injury although sometimes it could be difficult because the swelling, pain and muscle guarding. Lachman test is used to assess the anterior instability but it requires good muscle relaxation. It is usually performed at 20–30° of knee flexion. Stabilizing the distal femur with one hand and applying an anterior force to the proximal tibia with the other hand, the anterior laxity is assessed in the degree of anterior translation of the tibia. It should be compared with the contralateral knee. It has a sensitivity of 85 % and a specificity of 94 % for ACL ruptures [9].

The anterior draw test is similar to the Lachman, however, it is performed with the knee at 90 ° of flexion. It was only 41 % sensitive and 95 % specific [27].

Pivot shift test is performed applying slight distal traction on the leg, a valgus and internal rotation force to the extended knee. With maintenance of the forces noted above, the knee is then flexed past 30°. In an ACL deficient knee, in the intitial stages of knee flexion, the tibia will be anterolaterally subluxed on the distal femur with application of a valgus and internal rotation force at the knee. With further flexion of the knee (past approximately 30°), the iliotibial band goes from an extendor to a flexor of the knee and the tibial anterolateral subluxation reduces (shifts) back into place. Pivot Shift test has high specificity (98 %) in both acute and chronic conditions, but poor sensitivity (24 %) [27].

Imaging evaluation begins with plain film radiographs. On an anteroposterior view a tibial spine fracture that represents an avulsion of the ACL may be evident. Similarly, lateral capsule avulsion, a Segond fracture, is seen as a small vertical fracture at the lateral margin of the tibial plateau and is pathognomonic for an ACL disruption. In chronic injuries, one may see osteophyte formation, hypertrophy of the tibial spines, and joint space narrowing [7, 8].

Magnetic resonance imaging (MRI) is an invaluable test to the diagnosis of an ACL injury On T1 and T2 images, the normal ACL fibers can be visualized as they course from the tibial spine to the lateral femoral condyle. T1 images may demonstrate the absence of the normal fibers, while T2 images will demonstrate hemorrhage and edema within the injured ligament. MRI has a specificity of 95 % and a sensibility of 86 % for diagnosing ACL injuries, using arthroscopy as the gold standard [28]. MRI can also diagnose concomitant injuries such as meniscal tears, osteochondral defects, bone bruises, and other ligamentous injuries that may influence patient treatment [7] [8]. Geographic bone bruises are seen in more than 80 % of knees with acute ACL injuries. Most of these lesions will be in the posterior lateral tibial plateau and lateral femoral condyle. Patients usually have resolution of these bone bruises over several months, and they do not experience long-term consequences [29–32].

The KT1000 arthrometer is used to document abnormal anterior translation of the injured knee compared with the anterior translation of the normal knee preoperatively and in the postoperative period, to document surgical results instead of diagnosis in routine clinical practice.

10.5 Meniscal Injuries

In the ACL-defficient knee, the menisci act as an important secondary stabilizer to anterior translation [33]. Associated meniscus tears are relatively common in ACL injury. It is classically a vertical tear in either the medial or lateral meniscus within several millimeters of the peripheral rim where there is a blood supply to promote healing. Those that are less than 1–1.5 cm in length and that extend no more than halfway through the meniscus, do not need treatment. The tears that are posterior to the popliteus can be treated without resection and often do well [34]. Lateral meniscal tears are more common in acute injuries, occurring in 45–75 % of patients, while medial meniscal tears are more common in chronic injuries, occurring in 73–91 % of patients [35–39]. Nowadays, the recognition of the protective function of the meniscus has led to efforts to preserve as much meniscal tissue as possible. Numerous all-inside devices have been developed to facilitate meniscal repair performed entirely from within the joint. Meniscal repairs in an ACL reconstructed knee have a lower reoperation rate than isolated meniscal repairs, and that is even lower if the injury is in the lateral menisci. This may be related to the abundance of blood and growth factors in the joint, relatively limited patient activity and less aggressive rehabilitation after combined procedure and the intrinsic condition of the meniscus at the time of repair [40, 41].

10.6 Treatment

10.6.1 General Steps

Immediately after the injury patients should be advised to ice, compress, elevate and limit use of the knee (RICE).

10.6.2 Conservative Treatment/ Nonsurgical

This option consists in physical therapy aimed in getting a complete range of motion and strengthening the muscles around the knee, especially the quadriceps femoris and hamstring muscles. It could take until 6 months from the injury for muscles and neurologic control mechanisms to recover [42]. Nonsurgical treatment is indicated in patients that are not candidates for surgery because of serious comorbid medical conditions or patients whose surgery is not indicated due to a sedentary life style and asymptomatic with the daily activity.

10.6.3 Surgical Management

The goal when taking care of a patient with an ACL injury is to prevent recurrent injuries while allowing the patient to return to his/her desired level of work or sports.

Indications

- Patients with high level activity/athletes who practice sports or jobs with jumping, pivoting, hard cutting, e.g., basketball, football, and soccer. They will need an ACL reconstruction if they are to return to those [43].

- Symptomatic chronic ACL-deficient knees. Patiens that have returned to moderate activities after an ACL tear and have recurrent episodes of giving way, resulting in meniscus tears, pain, and repeated effusions.
- Special circumstances:
  - Patients with open physes, because children are inherently active and will damage their knees further if stability is not returned to the joint.
  - Those with persistent anterior knee pain after ACL injury that is related to quadriceps weakness and dynamic anterior tibial translation during activities. This latter motion can result in patellar tilt [44].
  - Patients with hypermobility: individuals in this group have lax secondary restraints that have large pivot-shift motions after the ACL is injured. This group will often have instability with even daily activities and will require surgical intervention [17].

Timing

Athletes often request early surgery to commence the rehabilitation process. Unfortunately, early surgery increases the risk of arthrofibrosis or stiffness and associated comorbidities including patellofemoral pain. In general, it takes at least 3 weeks for motion and quadriceps strength to return and truly 8 weeks for the knee to look close to normal. Full extension with a good quadriceps contraction and close to full flexion is desirable to do the reconstruction [17].

Although, a delay in surgical reconstruction could have a potential morbidity, such as inability to return to employment or sporting activities, as well as an increased risk of meniscal damage from further injuries [45], many surgeons prefer to treat injuries of the ACL 2 months or more after the injury, with an initial period of rehabilitation. This is because some studies have conclude that there is no advantage in early reconstruction for isolated tears of the ACL and that this is associated with an increased rate of complications, and delayed surgery is associated with a more rapid return of movement and muscle function [46, 47].

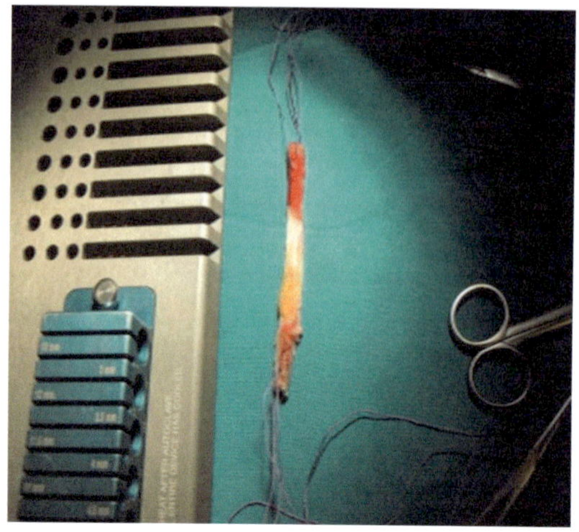

Fig. 10.1 The BTB (bone-tendon-bone) patellar tendon autograft

Graft Selection

The graft chosen should provide adequate fixation to allow rehabilitation, allow anatomic recreation of the ACL in both size and location and have adequate initial strength to survive the uncertainties of graft regeneration.

Patellar tendon graft

The central third patellar tendon, bone-tendon-bone graft (BTB) (Fig. 10.1) is the most commonly used graft in United States and is the gold standard. It is stiff and inelastic and, therefore, in theory, able to resist the high deforming forces in the unstable knee. The strength of graft fixation is also an important consideration and the bone plugs allow potentially very fast and secure bone-to-bone fixation in the bony tunnels [48]. The development by Kurosaka of interference screw fixation provides the strongest fixation available [49].

Although, being the gold standard, this graft has some light problems, mostly related to harvest. Anterior knee symptoms are common and have been reported in up to 80 % particularly with kneeling [50] for 6–9 months after surgery but only a relatively small percentage of patients consider that they have a significant problem [51]. The more serious complications could be the patellar tendon rupture and patellar fracture.

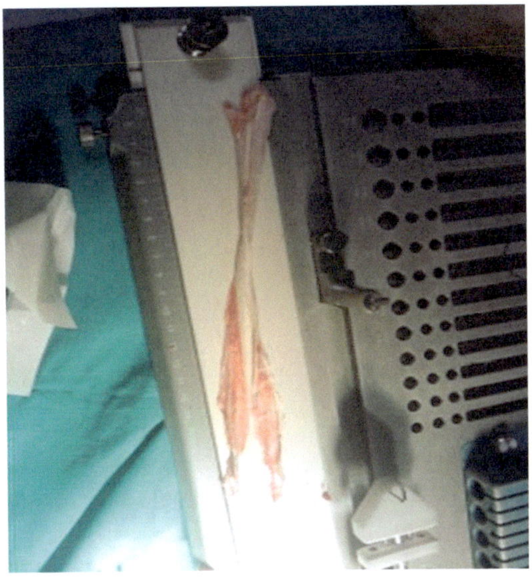

Fig. 10.2 Hamstring autograft before bending and tensioning

Quadriceps strength is impaired in virtually all ACL injured patients as a response to the loss of afferent nerves from the native ACL. Use of the patellar tendon graft accentuates this quadriceps atrophy, and it takes more than a year from surgery to regain close to normal strength [17]. Care should be taken to not overtension the graft and to place the knee in full extension at the time of fixation.

Hamstrings graft

Hamstring tendons (gracilis and semitendinosus tendons) (Fig. 10.2) were the first reported graft to reconstruct the ACL, and they continue to be a very popular graft [52, 53]. The size of the graft is related to the height, weight, and thigh circumference of the patient, and, although there is variability, four-strand grafts or double looped are virtually always between 7 and 10 mm in diameter [54]. A four-strand gracilis-semitendinosus graft functions better than a two-strand semitendinosus graft, but this necessitates tensioning all four strands equally at the time of fixation [55, 56]. Wilson et al., with their study of grafts confirmed that four-strand are significantly stronger than BTB patellar graft [57]. However, the risk of impingement is higher because of the larger size of the graft.

Postoperative soreness in the posterior thigh and lower leg in the first weeks after surgery can occur after hamstring harvest, but rarely for a long time. Clinically, patients feel their hamstring deficit has resolved by 4–6 months after reconstruction, but isokinetic testing will reveal slight deficits in knee flexion torque for up to 1 year, but a small loss of internal rotation torque can be measured because the muscles never reattach to the anteromedial tibia [58]. After harvesting the gracilis and semitendinosus tendons, MRI studies have documented healing of these muscles to the semimembranosus and posterior knee fascia.

Graft fixation has received a lot of attention of late, since fixing soft tissue to bone always provides more of a challenge than fixing bone-to-bone. At present, there are several options to choose, from double screws, cross-pin to interference screw and Endobutton. The last one is popular and the clinical results appear to be satisfactory [59, 60]. Soft tissue incorporation into the bone tunnels has been studied by Rodeo et al. in the dog [61] and it would appear that biological fixation occurs at a relatively early stage, between 8 and 12 weeks. In Table 10.1, we have summarised the differences between these two grafts.

Quadriceps tendon graft

A partial-thickness quadriceps tendon graft with or without a bone block from the proximal patella is another graft option. Unfortunately, there is some painful morbidity with use of this graft, and it has not become popular probably because of this fact [62]. If an autograft option is needed and the patellar tendon and hamstrings are not available, then this provides a good alternative.

Allograft

Allografts are an acceptable alternative to autografts [63]. With this graft there is less donor-side morbidity, availability of lager grafts, superior cosmesis, the possibility for multiple ligament reconstruction and operating times are reduced. However, the risk of disease transmission exists, although it is very, very small. The methods of sterilization available, irradiation and ethylene oxide significantly weaken the

Table 10.1 Advantages and disadvantages of patellar tendon grafts and hamstring grafts for ACL reconstruction

	Advantages	Disadvantages
Patella tendon grafts (gold standard)	• Excellent initial and long-term fixation (bone to bone) • Better overall stability/resistance	• Increased anterior knee pain • Quadriceps atrophy • Two incisions (plus arthroscopy portals)
Hamstring grafts	• 4-strand: very strong and resistant • Lower incidence of anterior knee pain and crepitus • Single incision (plus arthroscopy portals)	• Less secure initial and long-term fixation • Small loss in internal rotation torque • Impingement risk • Increased knee laxity after reconstruction

graft. Ethylene oxide is also considered to be responsible for cystic changes around the bone tunnels [48]. Another problem is that allografts heal more slowly than autografts do and they may have higher failures rates [64]. Because of that, surgeons usually slow the rehabilitation protocol when they are used. Tibialis tendon allograft is a good option. It needs smaller tunnels than BTB patellar tendon allograft and less concern about quality of bone plugs. The main indications for the use of allografts are in complex primary surgery or revision surgery.

Reconstruction Technique

In this section, we will discuss the most controversial aspects of the surgical technique.

• Notchplasty

The notchplasty provides several benefits as visualization of the ACL femoral attachment, prevention of graft impingement on the roof of the notch, and prevention of graft abrasion on the lateral wall of the notch [65, 66] Extending the knee while the notch is visualized provides a perspective on the potential for impingement and may direct the surgeon on how much bone to remove. Nevertheless, recent studies show that graft impingement might not happen in anatomical ACL reconstruction and because of that, notchplasty is not necessary in these cases [67].

• Tunnel placement

It is the critical key to ACL surgery. The tibial tunnel should exit on the tibial articular surface slightly medial to the anatomic center of the insertion site to prevent the graft from abrading on the lateral wall of the notch. The center of the tibial insertion should be approximately 15 mm anterior to the PCL notch, and the posterior border of the tunnel should be anterior to the peak of the medial tibial eminence [68]. The tunnel can be started just medial to the tibial tubercle where the bone quality is best and the drill guide angle chosen to create a tunnel that has a 30-mm minimum length. The angle should be of 60 or 65° with respect to the medial joint line of the tibia to decrease the risk of impingement.

Many studies emphasized the importance of femoral tunnel orientation to control anterior tibial translation and rotatory laxities [69–71]. Commonly used surgical technique of placing the graft in the femoral bone tunnel at the so-called 11 o'clock position in the right knee (and the 1 o'clock position in the left knee) replicates the anatomy of the anteromedial bundle, but not the posterolateral bundle, important for knee stabilization against rotational loads [72]. Because of that, internal rotation stability is not completely achieved. Thus, it has been proposed that a more horizontal placement (10 o'clock or 2 o'clock) of the graft can address abnormal rotational knee movement after a reconstruction of the ACL (anatomic position).

To locate the correct place, with the knee in 90° of flexion, two points are then identified: first, the apex of the notch, and second, the lowest point on the lateral wall. The point halfway between these two points is the anatomic center of the ACL. We may use an accessory anteromedial portal to drill it.

- Single bundle versus double bundle

The traditional surgical treatment for ACL rupture is arthroscopic single-bundle reconstruction. Nowadays, there is a tendency to use the double-bundle grafts that to more closely resemble the normal anatomy of the ACL by restoring the anteromedial (AM) and posterolateral (PL) bundles of the native ACL [73].

A recent meta-analysis says that there is insufficient evidence to determine the relative effectiveness of double-bundle and single-bundle reconstruction for anterior cruciate ligament rupture in adults, although there is limited evidence that double-bundle ACL reconstruction has some superior results in objective measurements of knee stability and protection against repeat ACL rupture or a new meniscal injury [74].

- Tensioning

Tensioning and fixation of the graft on the tibial side is critical and dependent on the type of graft, method of fixation, and laxity of the knee. Usually, fixation is done in flexion and the graft will lengthen with knee extension. In patellar tendon graft this does not happen because of the stiffness of the graft and they may not lengthen enough to allow extension. Therefore, it is suggested that patellar tendon grafts be tensioned and secured in close to full extension. Tensioning of multistranded grafts requires that all strands be tensioned equally to obtain the full strength of the graft [56].

Postoperative Management

The most important goals in the first week are controlling pain, swelling and inflammation, recovery of ROM (above all, full extension) and neuromuscular control [75, 76]. In addition to medication, exercises, postsurgical compression wraps and elevation, cryotherapy can reduce significantly postsurgical pain [77]. Bracing after surgery has not been shown to have an impact on results, but many surgeons use them [78, 79]. Crutches may be the best device to limit excessive activity in the first few weeks after surgery, promoting normal full knee extension and limiting excessive loads.

From the second week after surgery, quadriceps and hamstring strength can be increased by isometric isotonic and isokinetic exercises without endangering the graft. Specific exercises for this phase should include walking on a treadmill, cycling on an ergometer and swimming. Jogging and running can begin at 3–4 months based on the patient's progress, and full sports at 6 months [80].

10.7 Complications

Infection, deep vein thrombosis, loss of motion, patellofemoral pain, and general pain syndromes are the major complications that can significantly diminish the results of ACL surgery.

Postoperative septic arthritis is fortunately very uncommon with the routine preoperative antibiotics (typically a cephalosporin or clindamycin in allergic patients) with an incidence less than 1 % [81]. For treatment, experts recommend culture-specific antibiotics and surgical irrigation with graft retention as initial step. Graft and hardware removal are recommended only for persistent infection or an infected allograft [82]. The incidence of deep venous thrombosis and pulmonary embolism is very low, too. To prevent them early mobilization and compression device are used while routine porphylaxis remains controversial [83].

10.8 Conclusions

ACL surgery is indicated in active patients, with a high functional demand as well as in symptomatic patients with their usual activities. Early surgery can be associated with arthrofibrosis, stiffness and patellofemoral pain; because of that, surgery should be delayed until inflammation has disappeared. The gold standard of the grafts is the (BTB) patellar tendon autograft, but other options like hamstring tendons graft, quadriceps tendon graft or allografts have also good results. There are some controversial aspects in the reconstruction technique as the notchplasty that could provide benefits as visualization ACL femoral attachment, the tunnel placement that could increased the internal rotation stability, the use of single or double bundle or the best way of tensioning and fixation of the graft. Infection, deep vein thrombosis, loss of motion, patellofemoral pain, and general pain syndromes are the major complications, but fortunately are very uncommon. The incidence of infection is less than 1 % and it should be treated with culture-specific antibiotics and surgical irrigation.

References

1. Galen C (1968) On the usefulness of the parts of the body. May, MT (trans). Cornell University Press, Ithaca pp 22, 90, 151, 197, 550
2. Stark J (1850) Two cases of rupture of the crucial ligament of the knee-joint. Edinb Surg 74:267–271
3. Hey-Groves EW (1917) Operation for the repair of the crucial ligaments. Lancet 2:674–675
4. Odensten M, Gillquist J (1985) Functional anatomy of the anterior cruciate ligament and a rational for reconstruction. J Bone Joint Surg 67A:257–262
5. Girgis FG, Marshall JL, Monajem A (1975) The cruciate ligaments of the knee joint. Clin Orthop Relat Res 106:216–231
6. Harner CD, Baek GHB, Vogrin TM, Carlin GJ, Kashiwaguchi S, Woo SL (1999) Quantitative analysis of human cruciate ligament insertions. Arthroscopy 15:741–749
7. Daniel DM, Fritschy D (1994) Anterior cruciate ligament injuries. In: DeLee JC, Drez D Jr (eds) Orthopaedic sports medicine. Saunders, Philadelphia, pp 1313–1361
8. Wojtys EM (1994) The ACL deficient knee. American Academy of Orthopaedic Surgeons, Rosemont
9. Siegel L, Vandenakker-Albanese C, Siegel D (2012) Anterior cruciate ligament injuries: anatomy, physiology, biomechanics, and management. Clin J Sport Med 22(4):349–355 (review)
10. Khalfayan EE, Sharkey PF, Alexander AH, Bruckner JD, Bynum EB (1996) The relationship between tunnel placement and clinical results after anterior cruciate ligament reconstruction. Am J Sports Med 24:335–341
11. Yagi M, Wong EK, Kanamori A, Debski RE, Fu FH, Woo SL (2002) Biomechanical analysis of an anatomic anterior cruciate ligament reconstruction. Am J Sports Med 30:660–665
12. Yasuda K, Kondo E, Ichiyama H, Kitamura N, Tanabe Y, Tohyama J, Minami A (2004) Anatomic reconstruction of the anteromedial and posterolateral bundles of the anterior cruciate ligament using hamstring tendon grafts. Arthroscopy 20:1015–1025
13. Howell SM, Gittins ME, Gottlieb JE, Traina SM, Zoellner TM (2001) The relationship between the angle of the tibial tunnel in the coronal plane and loss of flexion and anterior laxity after anterior cruciate ligament reconstruction. Am J Sports Med 29:567–574
14. Heming JF, Rand J, Steiner ME (2007) Anatomic limitations of transtibial drilling in ACL reconstruction. Am J Sports Med 35:1708–1715
15. Mochizuki T, Muneta T, Nagase T, Shirawawa S, Akita K, Sekiya I (2006) Cadaveric knee observation study for describing anatomic femoral tunnel placement for two-bundle anterior cruciate ligament reconstruction. Arthroscopy 22:356–361
16. Morgan CD, Kalman KR, Grawl DM (1995) Definitive landmarks for reproducible tibial tunnel placement in anaterior cruciate ligament reconstruction. Arthroscopy 11:275–288
17. Steiner ME (2009) Surgical management of anterior cruciate ligament injuries. In: McKeon BP, Bono JV, Richmond JC (eds) Knee arthroscopy. Springer, New York, pp 129–152
18. Giuliani JR, Kilcoyne KG, Rue JP (2009) Anterior cruciate ligament anatomy: a review of the anteromedial and posterolateral bundles. J Knee Surg 22(2):148–154
19. Hootman JM, Dick R, Agel J (2007) Epidemiology of collegiate injuries for 15 sports: summary and recommendations for injury prevention initiatives. J Athl Train 42:311–319
20. Pujol N, Blanchi MP, Chambat P (2007) The incidence of anterior cruciate ligament injuries among competitive Alpine skiers: a 25-year investigation. Am J Sports Med 35:1070–1074
21. Anderson AF, Dome DC, Gautam S, Awh MH, Rennirt GW (2001) Correlation of anthropometric measurements, strength, anterior cruciate ligament size, and intercondylar notch characteristics to sex differences in anterior cruciate ligament tear rates. Am J Sports Med 29:58–66
22. Gwinn DE, Wilckens JH, McDevitt ER, Ross G, Kao TC (2000) The relative incidence of anterior cruciate ligament injury in men and women at the United States Naval Academy. Am J Sports Med 28:98–102
23. Arendt E, Dick R (1995) Knee injury patterns among men and women in collegiate basketball and soccer. NCAA data and review of literature. Am J Sports Med 23:694–701
24. Soprano JV (2005) Musculoskeletal injuries in the pediatric and adolescent athlete. Curr Sports Med Rep 4:329–334
25. Prodromos CC, Fu FH, Howell SM, Johnson DH, Lawhorn K (2008) Controversies in soft-tissue anterior cruciate ligament reconstruction: grafts, bundles, tunnels, fixation, and harvest. J Am Acad Orthop Surg 16:376–384

26. Boden BP, Torg JS, Knowles SB, Hewett TE (2009) Video analysis of anterior cruciate ligament injury: abnormalities in hip and ankle kinematics. Am J Sports Med 37:252–259
27. Katz JW, Fingeroth RJ (1986) The diagnostic accuracy of ruptures of the anterior cruciate ligament comparing the Lachman test, the anterior drawer sign, and the pivot shift test in acute and chronic knee injuries. Am J Sports Med 14(1):88–91
28. Spindler KP, Wright RW (2008) Clinical practice. Anterior cruciate ligament tear. N Engl J Med 359:2135–2142
29. Costa-Paz M, Muscolo D, Ayerza M, Makino A, Aponte-Tinao L (2001) Magnetic resonance imaging follow-up study of bone bruises associated with anterior cruciate ligament ruptures. Arthroscopy 17:445–449
30. Nakamae A, Engebretsen L, Bahr R, Krosshaug T, Ochi M (2006) Natural history of bone bruises after acute knee injury: clinical outcome and histopathological findings. Knee Surg Sports Traumatol Sports 14:1252–1258
31. Graf B, Cook D, De Smet A, Keene JS (1993) "Bone bruises" on magnetic resonance imaging evaluation of anterior cruciate ligament injuries. Am J Sports Med 21:220–223
32. Johnson D, Urban W, Caborn D, Vanarthos WJ, Carlson CS (1998) Articular cartilage changes seen with magnetic resonance imaging detected bone bruises associated with acute anterior cruciate ligament rupture. Am J Sports Med 26:409–414
33. Levy IM, Torzilli PA, Warren RF (1982) The effect of medial meniscectomy on anterior–posterior motion of the knee. J Bone Joint Surg 64A:883–888
34. Fitzgibbons R, Shelbourne KD (1995) "Aggressive" nontreatment of lateral meniscal tears seen during anterior cruciate ligament reconstruction. Am J Sports Med 23:156–159
35. Noyes FR, Bassett RW, Grood ES et al (1980) Arthroscopy in acute traumatic hemarthrosis of the knee: incidence of anterior cruciate tears and other injuries. J Bone Joint Surg 62A(5):687–695, 757
36. DeHaven KE (1980) Diagnosis of acute knee injuries with hemarthrosis. Am J Sports Med 8(1):9–14
37. Andersson C, Gillquist J (1992) Treatment of acute isolated and combined ruptures of the anterior cruciate ligament: a long-term follow-up study. Am J Sports Med 20:7–12
38. Fowler PJ, Regan WD (1987) The patient with symptomatic chronic anterior cruciate ligament insufficiency: results of minimal arthroscopic surgery and rehabilitation. Am J Sports Med 15:321–325
39. Indelicato PA, Bittar ES (1985) A perspective of lesions associated with ACL insufficiency of the knee: a review of 100 cases. Clin Orthop Relat Res 198:77–80
40. Schmitz MA, Rouse LM Jr, DeHaven KE (1996) The management of meniscal tears in the ACL-deficient knee. Clin Sports Med 15:573–593
41. Paxton ES, Stock MV, Brophy RH (2011) Meniscal repair versus partial meniscectomy: a systematic review comparing reoperation rates and clinical outcomes. Arthroscopy 27:1275–1288
42. Wojtys E, Huston L (1994) Neuromuscular performance in normal and anterior cruciate ligament-deficient lower extremities. Am J Sports Med 22:89–104
43. Feagin JA Jr, Curl WW (1976) Isolated tear of the anterior cruciate ligament: 5-year follow-up study. Am J Sports Med 4:95–100
44. Steiner M, Koskinen S, Winalski C et al (2001) Dynamic lateral patellar tilt in the ACL deficient knee. Am J Sports Med 29:593–599
45. Karlsson J, Kartus J, Magnusson L et al (1999) Subacute versus delayed reconstruction of the anterior cruciate ligament in the competitive athlete. Knee Surg Sports Traumatol Arthrosc 7:146–151
46. Shelbourne K, Wilckens JH, Mollabashy A, DeCarlo M (1991) Arthrofibrosis in acute anterior cruciate ligament reconstruction: the effect of timing of reconstruction and rehabilitation. Am J Sports Med 19:332–336
47. Peterson W, Laperell H (1999) Combined injuries of the medial collateral ligament and the anterior cruciate ligament: early ACL reconstruction versus late ACL reconstruction. Arch Orth Tr Surg 119:258–262
48. Allum RL (2001) BASK Instructional Lecture 1: graft selection in anterior cruciate ligament reconstruction. Knee 8:69–72
49. Kurosaka M, Yoshiya S, Andrish JT (1987) A biomechanical comparison of different surgical techniques of graft fixation in anterior cruciate ligament reconstruction. Am J Sports Med 15:225–229
50. Rosenberg TD, Franklin JL, Baldwin GN, Nelson KA (1992) Extensor mechanism function after patellar tendon graft harvest for anterior cruciate ligament reconstruction. Am J Sports Med 20:519–526
51. Burwell JMR, Davies AJ, Allum RL (1998) Anterior knee symptoms after reconstruction of the anterior cruciate ligament using patellar tendon as a graft. Knee 5:245–248
52. Hey-Groves WE (1920) The crucial ligaments of the knee joint: their function, rupture, and the operative treatment of the same. Br J Surg 7:505–515
53. Pinczewski P, Lyman J, Salmon L et al (2007) A 10-year comparison of anterior cruciate ligament reconstructions with hamstring tendon and patellar tendon autograft: a controlled, prospective trial. Am J Sports Med 35:564–574
54. Tuman J, Diduch D, Rubino L, Baumfeld JA, Nguyen HS, Hart JM (2007) Predictors for hamstring graft diameter in anterior cruciate ligament reconstruction. Am J Sports Med 35:1945–1949

55. Adachi N, Ochi M, Uchio Y, Iwasa J, Kuriwaka M, Ito Y (2004) Reconstruction of the anterior cruciate ligament single versus double bundle multistranded hamstring tendons. J Bone Joint Surg 86B:515–520
56. Hamner D, Brown C, Steiner M, Hecker AT, Hayes WC (1999) Hamstring tendon grafts for reconstruction of the anterior cruciate ligament: biomechanical evaluation of multiple strands and tensioning techniques. J Bone Joint Surg 81A:549–557
57. Wilson TW, Zafuta MP, Zobitz M (1999) A biomechanical analysis of matched bone-patellar tendon-bone and double-looped semitendinosus and gracilis tendon grafts. Am J Sports Med 27:202–207
58. Armour T, Forwell L, Litchfield R, Kirkley A, Amendola N, Fowler PJ (2004) Isokinetic evaluation of internal/external tibial rotation strength after the use of hamstring tendons for anterior cruciate ligament reconstruction. Am J Sports Med 32:1639–1643
59. Corry IS, Webb JM, Clingeleffer AJ, Pinczewski LA (1999) Arthroscopic reconstruction of the anterior cruciate ligament. A comparison of patellar tendon autograft and four-strand hamstring tendon autograft. Am J Sports Med 27:444–454
60. Jansson KA, Harilainen A, Sandelin J, Karjalainen PT, Aronen HJ, Tallroth K (1999) Bone tunnel enlargement after anterior cruciate ligament reconstruction with the hamstring autograft and endobutton fixation technique. A clinical, radiographic and magnetic resonance imaging study with 2 years follow up. Knee Surg Sports Traumatol Arthrosc 7:290–295
61. Rodeo SA, Arnoczky SP, Torzilli PA, Hidaka C, Warren RF (1993) Tendon-healing in a bone tunnel. A biomechanical and histological study in the dog. J Bone Joint Surg 75A:1795–1803
62. Adams D, Mazzocca A, Fulkerson J (2006) Residual strength of the quadriceps versus patellar tendon after harvesting a central free tendon graft. Arthroscopy 22:76–79
63. Harner CD, Olson E, Irrgang JJ, Silverstein S, Fu FH, Silbey M (1996) Allograft vs. autograft anterior cruciate ligament reconstruction: 3–5-year outcome. Clin Orth Relat Res 324:134–144
64. Ellis HB, Matheny LM, Briggs KK, Pennock AT, Steadman JR (2012) Outcomes and revision rate after bone-patellar tendon-bone allograft versus autograft anterior cruciate ligament reconstruction in patients aged 18 years or younger with closed physes. Arthroscopy 28: 1819-25
65. Muneta T, Yamamoto H, Ishibashi R, Asahina S, Murakami S, Furuya K (1995) The effects of tibial tunnel placement and roofplasty on reconstructed anterior cruciate ligament knees. Arthroscopy 11:57–62
66. Tanzer M, Lenczner E (1990) The relationship of intercondylar notch size and content to notchplasty requirement in anterior cruciate ligament surgery. Arthroscopy 6:89–93
67. Iriuchishima T, Shirakura K, Fu FH (2013) Graft impingement in anterior cruciate ligament reconstruction. Knee Surg Sports Traumatol Arthrosc 21: 664-70
68. Hantes M, Zachos V, Basdekis G, Zibis A, Dailiana Z, Malizos K (2006) Differences in graft orientation using the transtibial and anteromedial portal technique in ACL reconstruction: an MRI prospective study. J Bone Joint Surg Br 88(Suppl I):93
69. Loh JC, Fukuda Y, Tsuda E, Streadman RJ, Fu FH, Woo SL (2003) Knee stability and graft function following anterior cruciate ligament reconstruction: comparison between 11 o'clock and 10 o'clock femoral tunnel placement. Arthroscopy 19:297–304
70. Scopp JM, Jasper LE, Belkoff SM, Moorman CT 3rd (2004) The effect of oblique femoral tunnel placement on rotational constraint of the knee reconstructed using patellar tendon autografts. Arthroscopy 20(3):294–299
71. Yamamoto Y (2004) Knee stability and graft function after anterior cruciate ligament reconstruction. Am J Sports Med 32:1825–1832
72. Gabriel MT, Wong EK, Woo SL, Yagi M, Debski RE (2004) Distribution of in situ forces in the anterior cruciate ligament in response to rotatory loads. J Orthop Res 22:85–89
73. Odensten M, Gillquist J (1985) Functional anatomy of the anterior cruciate ligament and a rationale for reconstruction. J Bone Joint Surg Am 67:257–262
74. Tiamklang T, Sumanont S, Foocharoen T, Laopaiboon M (2012) Double-bundle versus single-bundle reconstruction for anterior cruciate ligament rupture in adults. Cochrane Database Syst Rev 11:CD008413
75. Cascio B, Culp L, Cosgarea A (2004) Return to play after anterior cruciate ligament reconstruction. Clin Sports Med 23:395–408
76. DeHaven K, Cosgarea A, Sebastianelli W (2003) Arthrofibrosis of the knee following ligament surgery. Instr Course Lect 52:369–381
77. Raynor M, Pietrobon R, Guller U, Higgins L (2005) Cryotherapy after ACL reconstruction. J Knee Surg 18:123–129
78. Harilainen A, Sandelin J (2006) Post-operative use of knee brace in bone-tendon-bone patellar tendon anterior cruciate ligament reconstruction, 5-year follow-up results of a randomized prospective study. Scand J Med Sci Sports 16:14–18
79. Henriksson M, Rockborn P, Good L (2002) Range of motion training in brace versus plaster immobilization after anterior cruciate ligament reconstruction, a prospective randomized comparison with a 2-year follow up. Scand J Med Sci Sports 12:73–80
80. Schmitt LC, Paterno MV, Hewett TE (2012) The impact of quadriceps femoris strength asymmetry on functional performance at return to sport following anterior cruciate ligament reconstruction. J Orthop Sports Phys Ther 42:750–759

81. Busam ML, Provencher MT, Bach BR Jr (2008) Complications of anterior cruciate ligament reconstruction with bone-patellar tendon-bone constructs: care and prevention. Am J Sports Med 36:379–394
82. Matava MJ, Evans TA, Wright RW, Shively RA (1998) Septic arthritis of the knee following anterior cruciate ligament reconstruction: results of a survey of sports medicine fellowship directors. Arthroscopy 14:717–725
83. Cullison TR, Muldoon MP, Gorman JD, Goff WB (1996) The incidence of deep venous thrombosis in anterior cruciate ligament reconstruction. Arthroscopy 12:657–659

11 Runner's Knee and Patellar Tendinopathy

E. Carlos Rodríguez-Merchán, Hortensia De la Corte-García, Hortensia De la Corte-Rodríguez and Juan Manuel Román-Belmonte

11.1 Introduction

Patellofemoral pain syndrome (PFPS) , also known as runner's knee, is a common cause of anterior knee pain in young active recreational and professional athletes. The prevalence of PFPS in the general population is 1–4 % [1], and 20–25 % of all running injuries that present at sports medicine clinics are diagnosed as PFPS [2–4]. Besides runners, PFPS also occurs in soccer, hockey and volleyball players. It has been reported that PFPS secondary to patellar tendinopathy (PT) affects nearly 50 % of all top volleyball players [5].

The clinical presentation of PFPS is characterized by pain behind and around the patella, which intensifies with running, prolonged sitting, squatting, and ascending and descending stairs [6]. The pathogenesis of PFPS remains unclear and its etiology is multi-factorial. Diagnostic radiological imaging often fails to detect specific findings [7]. There is no consensus in the literature on the best conservative treatment to treat PFPS secondary to PT. Nor is there agreement on what surgical procedure is most appropriate when non-surgical treatment fails [8, 9]. The purpose of this review chapter is to discuss the strategies available for conservative and surgical treatment of PFPS and PT.

A search of English-language papers published until 2012 was conducted to look for references to PFPS and PT. Thirty-seven papers were selected for this study. The quality of the articles chosen was determined on the basis on the authors' judgment. Articles were included if they specifically addressed the treatment of PFPS and PT.

Both PFPS and PT often lead to considerable functional disability in recreational as well as professional athletes [10]. These conditions can interfere with sports performance, persist throughout an athlete's sporting career and even result in a premature end to a career in sports. The diagnosis of PFPS and PT is mainly based on clinical findings although new imaging technologies such as doppler ultrasonography may also be of diagnostic value, particularly in cases of PT. Two main strategies exist for

E. C. Rodríguez-Merchán (✉)
Department of Orthopaedic Surgery, "La Paz" University Hospital-IdiPaz, Paseo de la Castellana 261, 28046, Madrid, Spain
e-mail: ecrmerchan@gmx.es

H. De la Corte-García · J. M. Román-Belmonte
Department of Physical Medicine and Rehabilitation, "Doce de Octubre" University Hospital, Avenida de Córdoba S/N, 28041, Madrid, Spain
e-mail: hortensia.corte@yahoo.es

J. M. Román-Belmonte
e-mail: calamaris18@hotmail.com

H. De la Corte-Rodríguez
Department of Physical Medicine and Rehabilitation, "La Paz" University Hospital, Paseo de la Castellana 261, 28046, Madrid, Spain
e-mail: hortensiadelacorterodriguez@yahoo.es

E. C. Rodríguez-Merchán (ed.), *Traumatic Injuries of the Knee*,
DOI: 10.1007/978-88-470-5298-7_11, © Springer-Verlag Italia 2013

treatment of PFPS and PT: conservative treatment and surgical treatment.

11.2 Conservative Treatment

The main non-surgical strategies for the management of runner's knee and PT are physical therapy, patellar taping and foot orthoses, extracorporeal shockwave therapy (ESWT), and injection treatments (dry needling, autologous blood, high-volume fluid therapy, platelet-rich plasma concentrate, sclerosis, steroids, aprotinin injections, ultrasound-guided injection of autologous skin-derived tendon-like cells and inoculation of bone marrow mononuclear cells).

11.2.1 Physiotherapy

PPS can be treated by patellar mobilization. The results of a systematic review showed that the combination of quadriceps strengthening exercises with hip strengthening exercises is a useful treatment strategy [11]. Biofeedback, patella taping, and foot orthoses may augment the benefits gained from quadriceps exercises [11]. Open and closed kinetic chain exercises have been shown to be equally effective [12]. Ultrasound therapy has shown itself to have a beneficial effect in terms of relieving the pain caused by PPS [13]. Direct application of adhesive medical tape to the skin around the patella relieves pain and ameliorates function even if its longer-term effects are uncertain. Nonetheless, the data provided by existing studies do adequately characterize the merits of taping, whether used on its own or as part of a more comprehensive treatment program [14].

11.2.2 Patella Taping and Foot Orthoses

Patella taping and foot orthoses may augment the benefits gained from quadriceps exercises. Application of orthotic devices e.g. knee braces, knee straps, different forms of tapes and bandages, active training equipment, compression sleeves and arch support insoles has been recommended as treatment for patellofemoral pain syndrome. Moreover, foot orthoses may provide short-term pain relief [15]. It must be added, however, that the number of randomized controlled studies carried out so far is still too low to warrant any firm conclusions about the efficacy of knee and foot orthotics in the treatment of patellofemoral pain [16].

11.2.3 Extracorporeal Shockwave Therapy (ESWT)

Since the initial studies on the efficacy of ESWT [17], several reports have shown that shock waves are effective in the treatment of chronic PT. In 2007 Van Leeuwen et al. [18] reviewed the existing literature on chronic PT. With a maximum follow-up of 36 months, these authors found that ESWT relieved pain and improved function. In a randomized study, Zwerver et al. [19] compared ESWT versus placebo in patients with symptoms of PT of 3–12 months' duration. They only a subjective improvement for ESWT. Recent reports show that ESWT could have a chondroprotective effect on the knee [20], and also that it could prevent progression of osteoarthritis [21, 22]. Over the last few years ESWT has become an excellent technique for the treatment of musculoskeletal problems that fail to respond to initial non-surgical treatment. Given that adverse effects and complications of ESWT are minimal, shock waves are considered safe and effective in the treatment of chronic PT [23, 24].

11.2.4 Injection Treatments

Injection treatments have become increasingly common in the treatment of PFPS secondary to PT. Van Ark et al. [25] described seven types of injection treatment (dry needling, autologous blood, high-volume fluid therapy, platelet-rich plasma, sclerosis, steroids and aprotinin injections) together with their rationale and effectiveness. All seven injection treatments exhibited promising results for the treatment of PT. Unlike other injection treatments, steroid treatment often showed a recurrence of symptoms in the long term. Caution must be exercised in analyzing the results as the number of studies reviewed was low, their quality was in some cases questionable and the methodology used in them was not always the same, which makes them difficult to compare.

Clarke et al. [26] compared the effectiveness of ultrasound-guided injection of autologous skin-derived tendon-like cells with that of other types of injection treatments in patients with refractory PFPS. These authors used skin biopsies from 60 patellar tendons in 46 patients with intractable PT to grow tenocyte-like collagen-producing cells. Patients were randomized into receiving an injection of either dermal fibroblast-derived amplified collagen-producing cells suspended in autologous plasma from autologous whole blood; or autologous plasma alone. Injections were applied to sites where hypoechogenicity, intrasubstance tears or fibrillar patellar tendon damage were observed. Ultrasound-guided injection of autologous skin-derived tendon-like cells exhibited a faster therapeutic effect and a significantly greater improvement in pain and function than with plasma alone.

Pascual-Garrido et al. [27] treated eight patients with chronic PT by means of inoculation of bone marrow mononuclear cells (BM-MNCs). According to their results, inoculation of BM-MNCs could be considered a potentially effective therapy for patients with chronic PT refractory to non-surgical treatment.

11.3 Surgical Treatment

Surgical treatment of runner's knee and patellar tendinopathy can be performed either by open surgery or by arthroscopy.

11.3.1 Open Surgical Treatment

Ferreti et al. [28] performed a retrospective study to analyze the results of surgical treatment in competitive athletes with patellar tendinopathy. Their cohort comprised 32 patients (38 knees) treated surgically following failure of conservative treatment. The surgical technique used included the following steps: longitudinal splitting of the tendonlongitudinal splitting of the tendon, resection of any pathological tissue encountered and patellar drilling through Hoffa's fat pad. Long-term results were good or excellent in 28 knees (83 %). Eighty-two percentage of the patients were able to pursue sports at their preinjury level, with 63 % of those knees being totally symptom-free. The results were less predictable in volleyball players.

Tendonectomy (surgical removal of necrotic tissue), surgical stimulation of the remaining tendon and specific aggressive postoperative rehabilitation have been found to be safe and effective in returning high-level athletes to their previous sports [29]. Kaeding et al. found a 71 % success rate when surgical treatment of the inferior pole of the patella was performed compared to 92 % when no patella bony work was carried out. Closure of the paratenon showed an 85 % success rate compared to 91.5 % when no paratenon closure was performed. Immobilization showed an 82.5 % success rate compared to a 95 % success rate when no postoperative immobilization was indicated.

11.3.2 Arthroscopic Treatment

A new arthroscopic approach based on imaging findings reported by Willberg et al. has yielded promising short-term results [30]. The authors included fifteen patients (15 knees) with a diagnosis of runner's knee or patellar tendinopathy. All patients had long-standing pain related to the patellar tendon (mean: 27 months). Ultrasonography plus color doppler examination showed structural changes and hypo-echoic areas and neovascularization inside the tendon and on its dorsal aspect, which corresponded to the painful area. All patients underwent arthroscopic shaving of the dorsal side of the proximal tendon, which centered mainly on the area where neovessels and nerves were located. The procedure succeeded in reducing tendon pain and allowed the majority of patients to go back to full tendon loading within 2 months after surgery.

Ogon et al. described a different arthroscopic technique for the treatment of chronic patellar tendinopathy [31]. The technique consisted in arthroscopically removing any hypertrophic synovitis from the inferior patellar pole. Two outside-in cannulas located between the tendon insertion site and the lateral aspect of the patellar tendon were used to mark the symptomatic region. A bipolar cautery was used to release the paratenon and denervate the inferior pole of the patella, including the tendon attachment site within the marked area. As no tendon or bone material was removed or excised throughout the procedure, the tendon was subjected to minimal surgical impact, which allowed an early and functional rehabilitation. The technique was effective, easy to perform, and safe to apply.

Kelly examined the results of arthroscopically debriding the patellar tendon and resecting the inferior pole of the patella in patients with refractory patellar tendinopathy [32]. He concluded that arthroscopic excision of the distal patellar pole with tendon débridement held promise for the treatment of intractable patellar tendinopathy. Lorbach et al. performed a prospective study to evaluate the clinical results of arthroscopic resection of the lower patellar pole in patients with patellar tendinopathy [33] and observed that the technique was effective in improving knee function and resulted in significant pain relief, which allowed patients prompt resumption of sport activity.

Pascarella et al. [34] conducted a study of 64 patients (73 knees), subjected to arthroscopy for patellar tendinopathy following the failure of non-surgical management. All 64 patients, 27 of whom were professional athletes, underwent arthroscopic débridement of the fat pad located behind the patellar tendon, débridement of any pathologic tendon tissue and resection of the distal patella. All patients were able to return to sports within 3 months. Arthroscopic surgery for patellar tendinopathy refractory to non-surgical management appeared to provide a significant improvement in terms of symptoms and function. This improvement persisted for at least 3 years. Nevertheless, not all patients were able to regain their preinjury sporting level and those who resumed sports practice did so with some degree of residual symptoms.

11.4 Comparative Studies

Willberg et al. [35] compared the after-treatment clinical effects of sclerosing polidocanol injections and arthroscopic shaving. Patients treated with arthroscopic shaving had significantly less pain at rest and during activity, and were significantly more satisfied compared with patients in the sclerosing injection group. Both ultrasound and color doppler-guided sclerosing polidocanol injections and arthroscopic shaving showed good clinical results, but patients treated with the latter had less pain and were more satisfied with the results of treatment. Cucurulo et al. reported that arthroscopic techniques seemed to be as effective as open surgery with an equivalent time to resumption of sports activity [36]. Surgical treatment was compared with eccentric training by Bahr et al. [37], who found no advantages of surgery over eccentric strength training. However, the same authors point out that eccentric training should be attempted for 12 weeks before considering surgery for the treatment of patellar tendinopathy.

11.5 Conclusions

There is moderate evidence that intrinsic risk factors may influence patellofemoral joint loading, resulting in potential muscle imbalances and biomechanical alterations and contributing to the onset of pain. Extrinsic risk factors such as poor training habits and improper footwear may also lead to patellofemoral pain. To avoid injuries, total weekly running distance should not exceed 64 km. There is high-quality evidence indicating an association between running-related lower limb injuries and training volume [6]. Patients developing PFPS during adolescence have a better prognosis, with their symptoms tending to resolve spontaneously (moderate level of evidence).

In adults with PFPS, intensive quadriceps rehabilitation is required if symptoms do not resolve spontaneously (moderate level of evidence).

The combination of quadriceps strengthening exercises with hip strengthening exercises has proved useful in the treatment of PFPS secondary to patellar tendinopathy. On the other hand, patella taping and foot orthoses may augment the benefits gained from quadriceps exercise. There is strong evidence that open and closed kinetic chain exercises are equally effective. Injection treatments (dry needling, autologous blood, high-volume fluid therapy, platelet-rich plasma, sclerosis, steroids and aprotinin injections) are increasingly used as treatment for PFPS secondary to patellar tendinopathy. ESWT is a safe and effective technique for the treatment of chronic patellar tendinopathy.

Surgical treatment of PFPS secondary to patellar tendinopathy must be indicated in motivated athletes if carefully followed non-surgical treatment is unsuccessful after 3–6 months, preventing them from returning to sports practice [38]. Arthroscopic techniques seem to be as effective as open surgery. They include arthroscopic shaving of the dorsal side of the proximal tendon, removal of the hypertrophic synovitis around the inferior patellar pole and arthroscopic tendon débridement with excision of the distal pole of the patella.

References

1. McConnell JJ (1986) The management of chnodromalacia patellae: a long-term solution. Aust J Physiother 32:215–223
2. Taunton JE, Ryan MB, Clement DB et al (2002) A retrospective case-control analysis of 2002 running injuries. Br J Sports Med 36:95–101
3. Pinshaw R, Atlas V, Nokaes TD (1984) The nature and response to therapy of 196 consecutive injuries seen at a runnerś clinic. S Afr Med 65:291–298
4. Ballas MT, Tytko J, Cookson D (1997) Common overuse running injuries: diagnosis and management. Am Fam Physician 55:2473–2484
5. Hyman GS (2008) Jumper's knee in volleyball athletes: advancements in diagnosis and treatment. Curr Sports Med Rep 7:296–302
6. Mears SC, Cosgarea AJ (2001) Surgical treatment options in patellofemoral disorders. Curr Opin Orthop 12:167–173
7. Yeung EW, Yeung SS (2002) Runnerś knee. In: Bhandari M (ed) Evidence-based Orthopedics. Wiley-Blackwell, Oxford, pp 853–859
8. Rees JD, Maffulli N, Cook J (2009) Management of tendinopathy. Am J Sports Med 37:1855–1867
9. Kaeding CC, Pedroza AD, Powers BC (2007) Surgical treatment of chronic patellar tendinosis: a systematic review. Clin Orthop Relat Res 455:102–106
10. Peers KH, Lysens RJ (2005) Patellar tendinopathy in athletes: current diagnostic and therapeutic recommendations. Sports Med 35:71–78
11. Bolgla LA, Boling MC (2011) An update for the conservative management of patellofemoral pain syndrome: a systematic review of the literature from 2000 to 2010. Int J Sports Phys Ther 6:112–125
12. Heintjes E, Berger MY, Bierma-Zeinstra SM, Bernsen RM, Verhaar JA, Koes BW (2003) Exercise therapy for patellofemoral pain syndrome. Cochrane Database Syst Rev (4):CD003472
13. Brosseau L, Casimiro L, Robinson V, Milne S, Shea B, Judd M, Wells G, Tugwell P (2001) Therapeutic ultrasound for treating patellofemoral pain syndrome. Cochrane Database Syst Rev (4):CD003375
14. Callaghan MJ, Selfe J (2012) Patellar taping for patellofemoral pain syndrome in adults. Cochrane Database Syst Rev (4):CD006717
15. Hossain M, Alexander P, Burls A, Jobanputra P (2011) Foot orthoses for patellofemoral pain in adults. Cochrane Database Syst Rev 19(1):CD008402
16. D'hondt NE, Struijs PA, Kerkhoffs GM, Verheul C, Lysens R, Aufdemkampe G, Van Dijk CN (2009) Orthotic devices for treating patellofemoral pain syndrome. Cochrane Database Syst Rev (1):CD002267
17. Wen-Wei HS, Hsu WH, Tai CL, Lee KF (2004) Effect of shock-wave therapy on patellar tendinopathy in a rabbit model. J Orthop Res 1:221–227
18. van Leeuwen MT, Zwerver J, van den Akker-Scheek I (2009) Extracorporeal shockwave therapy for patellar tendinopathy: a review of the literature. Br J Sports Med 43:163–168
19. Zwerver J, Hartgens F, Verhagen E, van der Worp H, van den Akker-Scheek I, Diercks RL (2011) No effect of extracorporeal shockwave therapy on patellar tendinopathy in jumping athletes during the competitive season: a randomized clinical trial. Am J Sports Med 39:1191–1199
20. Wang CJ, Sun YC, Wong T, Hsu SL, Chou WY, Chang HW (2012) Extracorporeal shockwave therapy shows time-dependent chondroprotective effects in osteoarthritis of the knee in rats. J Surg Res 178:196–205
21. Wang CJ, Weng LH, Ko JY, Sun YC, Yang YJ, Wang FS (2011) Extracorporeal shockwave therapy shows chondroprotective effects in osteoarthritic rat knee. Arch Orthop Trauma Surg 131:1153–1158
22. Wang CJ, Weng LH, Ko JY, Wang JW, Chen JN, Sun YC, Yang YJ (2011) Extracorporeal shockwave shows regression of osteoarthritis of the knee in rats. J Surg Res 171:601–608

23. Wang CJ (2012) Extracorporeal shockwave therapy in musculoskeletal disorders. J Orthop Surg Res 7:11
24. Wang CJ, Ko JY, Chan YS, Weng LH, Hsu SL (2007) Extracorporeal shockwave for chronic patellar tendinopathy. Am J Sports Med 35:972–978
25. van Ark M, Zwerver J, van den Akker-Scheek I (2011) Injection treatments for patellar tendinopathy. Br J Sports Med 45:1068–1076
26. Clarke AW, Alyas F, Morris T, Robertson CJ, Bell J, Connell DA (2011) Skin-derived tenocyte-like cells for the treatment of patellar tendinopathy. Am J Sports Med 39:614–623
27. Pascual-Garrido C, Rolón A, Makino A (2012) Treatment of chronic patellar tendinopathy with autologous bone marrow stem cells: a 5-year-follow-up. Stem Cells Int 953510
28. Ferretti A, Conteduca F, Camerucci E, Morelli F (2002) Patellar tendinosis: a follow-up study of surgical treatment. J Bone Joint Surg Am 84-A:2179–2185
29. Shelbourne KD, Henne TD, Gray T (2006) Recalcitrant patellar tendinosis in elite athletes: surgical treatment in conjunction with aggressive postoperative rehabilitation. Am J Sports Med 34:1141–1146
30. Willberg L, Sunding K, Ohberg L, Forssblad M, Alfredson H (2007) Treatment of Jumper's knee: promising short-term results in a pilot study using a new arthroscopic approach based on imaging findings. Knee Surg Sports Traumatol Arthrosc 15:676–681
31. Ogon P, Maier D, Jaeger A, Suedkamp NP (2006) Arthroscopic patellar release for the treatment of chronic patellar tendinopathy. Arthroscopy 22(462):e1–e5
32. Kelly JD 4th (2009) Arthroscopic excision of distal pole of patella for refractory patellar tendinitis. Orthopedics 32:504
33. Lorbach O, Diamantopoulos A, Paessler HH (2008) Arthroscopic resection of the lower patellar pole in patients with chronic patellar tendinosis. Arthroscopy 24:167–173
34. Pascarella A, Alam M, Pascarella F, Latte C, Di Salvatore MG, Maffulli N (2011) Arthroscopic management of chronic patellar tendinopathy. Am J Sports Med 39:1975–1983
35. Willberg L, Sunding K, Forssblad M, Fahlström M, Alfredson H (2011) Sclerosing polidocanol injections or arthroscopic shaving to treat patellar tendinopathy/jumper's knee? A randomised controlled study. Br J Sports Med 45:411–415
36. Cucurulo T, Louis ML, Thaunat M, Franceschi JP (2009) Surgical treatment of patellar tendinopathy in athletes. A retrospective multicentric study. Orthop Traumatol Surg Res 95(8 Suppl 1):S78–S84
37. Bahr R, Fossan B, Løken S, Engebretsen L (2006) Surgical treatment compared with eccentric training for patellar tendinopathy (Jumper's Knee). A randomized, controlled trial. J Bone Joint Surg Am 88:1689–1698
38. Rodríguez-Merchán EC (2012) The treatment of patellar tendinopathy. J Orthop Traumatol. [Epub ahead of print]

Index

E. C. Rodríguez-Merchán (ed.), *Traumatic Injuries of the Knee*,
DOI: 10.1007/978-88-470-5298-7, © Springer-Verlag Italia 2013

MIX
Papier aus verantwortungsvollen Quellen
Paper from responsible sources
FSC® C105338

If you have any concerns about our products,
you can contact us on
ProductSafety@springernature.com

In case Publisher is established outside the EU,
the EU authorized representative is:
Springer Nature Customer Service Center GmbH
Europaplatz 3, 69115 Heidelberg, Germany

Printed by Libri Plureos GmbH
in Hamburg, Germany